The Patient and
the Plastic Surgeon

The Patient and the Plastic Surgeon

ROBERT M. GOLDWYN, M.D.

Clinical Professor of Surgery, Harvard Medical School; Head, Division of Plastic Surgery, Beth Israel Hospital; Surgeon, Beth Israel Hospital and Brigham and Women's Hospital, Boston; Editor, Plastic and Reconstructive Surgery

Little, Brown and Company, Boston

Library of Congress Catalog Card No. 81-81009
ISBN 0-316-31974-0
Printed in the United States of America
MV

TO MY MOTHER AND FATHER
fortunatus fui

Contents

Preface

I have written this book to share my observations and thoughts with other plastic surgeons. It is a personal statement about taking care of patients, not a manual on office procedure or an encyclopedia on the doctor–patient relationship. Library shelves already buckle from the latter, which recently have come mostly from nonmedical authors. Of physicians writing on this topic, few have been plastic surgeons. Although what transpires between patient and plastic surgeon has many similarities with other doctor-patient relationships, there are differences that are crucial to recognize and to act upon. I hope this book will aid in the care of patients by increasing the awareness of the dynamics and subtleties in the interaction between patient and plastic surgeon, particularly during the initial consultation. For most of us, helping people was the stimulus that prompted our choosing medicine as a career, that buoyed us during the troughs of medical school and residency, and that still occupies most of our waking and working lives.

By examining the role of the doctor and the patient, this book emphasizes the actions and reactions of each and the effects and consequences for both. As a physician, I was conscious of the temptation to confine my sights mostly to the patient. This narrowness of focus, however, has been the defect of other writings on this subject. We must not forget that when we do something to a patient, we are doing something also to ourselves and the patient is doing something to us.

Medicine has survived because humankind is subject to disease and death. That one person has a problem and that another might have a solution is the immutable crux of the singular alliance between doctor and patient.

Finally, for humility and balance, we should remember that we who are physicians will eventually become patients. While it may be impossible to establish the priority between chicken and egg, it is certain that there was disease before there was medicine, and there were patients before there were doctors.

R. M. G.

Acknowledgments

Readers will recognize the influences of many in the writing of this book. I have recorded consciously and unconsciously the experience and wisdom of past and present teachers, colleagues, friends, and, particularly, patients. To all of them I am grateful. In addition, I wish to thank those who read the manuscript at different stages: Henry U. Grunebaum, M.D.; Judith Grunebaum, M.S.W.; S. Michael Kalick, Ph.D.; Estrellita Karsh; and my wife, Roberta. Their suggestions significantly improved the book.

I continue to benefit from the support and skills of my publishers: Fred Belliveau, Vice President and General Manager of the Medical Division of Little, Brown and Company, and Jane Mac-Neil, project editor *extraordinaire*. I am grateful also to copyeditor Judy Jamison-Perkins, proofreader Cecilia Thurlow, and indexer Patricia Perrier for their talents and dedication.

Bobbi Quigley, my secretary, with her customary competence and cheerfulness, once again typed the many drafts of this manuscript. Patricia G. Reilly helped with the final product.

My gratitude also to Kate Belmonte, who verified all references.

I appreciate the willingness of my colleagues to allow me to reproduce their patient information sheets: James L. Baker, Jr., M.D.; Frederick M. Grazer, M.D.; Bernard L. Kaye, M.D., D.M.D.; John G. Penn, M.D.; Thomas D. Rees, M.D.; and John E. Williams, M.D.

The great thing is to last and get your work done and see and hear and learn and understand; and write when there is something that you know; and not before; and not too damned much after.
ERNEST HEMINGWAY
Death in the Afternoon

Illness is the night-side of life, a more onerous citizenship. Everyone who was born holds dual citizenship in the kingdom of the well and in the kingdom of the sick. Although we all prefer to use only the good passport, sooner or later each of us is obliged, at least for a spell, to identify ourselves as citizens of that other place.
SUSAN SONTAG
Illness as Metaphor

*The Patient and
the Plastic Surgeon*

1. The Initial Consultation: Concepts and Components

He was a 20-year-old black from Mississippi; he had left the state that summer for the first time to attend the Harvard Health Professions Program, which enables minority students to view firsthand the workings of medicine. After a morning with me in the operating room and a long afternoon at the office, he exclaimed enthusiastically to his weary mentor, "It must be wonderful having people come to you for help and being able to take care of them." With his unfettered wisdom, he had captured the essence of medicine, which too often is lost in the process of doctoring. But what this young man just beginning his arduous medical journey did not realize was that the patient with treatable ills and the physician with ample skills do not necessarily equal a happy outcome. When and why things go right between patient and plastic surgeon and when and why they go wrong are what this book is about.

At what point in life does a plastic surgeon's occupation become "plastic surgeon" instead of "surgeon" or "physician"? I am conscious of these choices whenever I must declare myself, as, for example, when registering at a hotel. I am haunted by that sad, perhaps apocryphal, epitaph: "Here Lies _____. Born a Man, Died a Gastroenterologist." It would be interesting to poll the approximately 2,000 board-certified plastic surgeons of the United States, asking what they consider themselves to be: physician, surgeon, or plastic surgeon. The question is not trivial, since each response probably reflects different attitudes about what he thinks of himself and what he thinks his relationship to the patient is or should be. My personal concept is that I am first a physician and second a plastic surgeon. Somehow, despite my five years of training and board certification in general surgery, I do not picture myself primarily as a surgeon in the generic sense, but as something even broader—physician; and more specifically—plastic surgeon.

Whatever our professional self-image, it is apt to be blurred by the influx of patients and the daily demands of their management.

So complex has the edifice of medicine become that the cornerstone, the interaction between patient and doctor, has been hidden from view. Talking about the physician and the patient is usually reserved for graduation day—in a speech given by those who do not have their own patients. A worried premedical student asked me whether, when he went for his medical school interview, he should admit that he wanted to become a doctor because he hoped to help people. He was afraid that this sentiment would sound false. I told him to say what he believed; truly his motivation was not shameful for a would-be doctor.

The cynicism of our age has made us distrust those who say that they love their parents, trust their leaders, and enjoy their bond with their patients. As one young resident observed, "Love and compassion are relevant dimensions in the whole doctor-patient relationship. Somehow, this is never mentioned on the ward. Ever [149]."

But what is this relationship?

The Relationship Between Physician and Patient

The phrase *doctor-patient relationship*, albeit worn, still denotes a special interaction. Although it has been called a "two-party contract," it contains much that is noncontractual—intangibles that cannot be guaranteed in any legal agreement between two people [95, 109–111]. Indeed, the confusion in the doctor-patient interchange relates to these impalpable but critical components of concern and compassion. In general, patients desire more than having a service performed. Seneca, the Roman statesman and philosopher, wrote: "If, therefore, a physician does nothing more than feel my pulse and put me on the list of those whom he visits on his rounds, instructing me what to do and what to avoid without any personal feeling, I owe him nothing more than his fee, because he does not see me as a friend but as a client [128]." Seneca had in mind this quality of caring on the part of the physician, not just technical competence meted out perfunctorily.

So long have human beings endured pain and disease that all societies have developed specific expectations of behavior from those who are ill and from those who are supposed to treat them

[40, 83]. Being sick has its role requirements, as does being well [88, 124, 132].

In all cultures, the one who is ill has a responsibility to help himself get better with guidance from the healer, who is the physician in our society. While sickness is allowed, under most circumstances it is not praised or perpetuated since no society could function effectively or survive if most of its members were unable to perform their tasks, such as gathering food, bearing children, and defending the community.

In general, a patient consults a doctor because of a problem, real or imagined, and the need for help. Few patients have the competence to make a medical decision or the means to implement it. They are likely to be under strain—emotional, physical, or both. They hope that their problem is not serious, that recovery will be rapid, and that medical care will be affordable.

No office with honor is without onus, and that of the healer is no exception. For the privilege and power bestowed by the culture, the healer has definite responsibilities to the sick. These include being available, utilizing maximally his or her skills to help the patient, and behaving with concern, compassion, dignity, and honesty. The healer must not exploit the patient, sexually, financially, or in any other way.

In a world with so much mistrust, it is reassuring and even surprising to witness how patients will reveal confidences, allow examination (and even photographs) of parts of the body usually not seen by strangers, entrust their lives to a person known to them just a few minutes before only by name; sometimes, as in emergencies, even that is unknown. The success of this process is facilitated by a secure childhood for both patient and doctor in terms of rewarding, unbetraying relationships, and is due not just to the performance of that doctor or patient during the initial consultation but also to centuries of successful doctor–patient interactions. Any erosion of that trust has consequences not just for a particular patient and doctor but for future patients and physicians. Faith in proper enactment of roles is not unique to medicine or our society or our times. It has existed whenever and wherever living has become sufficiently complex to require different tasks of different people. In small, primitive societies, entrusting one's life to an unknown human being is rare. In our culture it is commonplace. We allow restaurants (unseen cooks) to prepare our meals and, as air passengers, we put our lives in the hands of pilots whom we have never met and trust machinery that we cannot understand.

SELFISHNESS AND ALTRUISM

To think of the physician and the practice of medicine as being "altruistic" and of some other activities of our society, such as business, as being "selfish" would be naive and incorrect. Parsons noted: "the seeming paradox is . . . that it is to a physician's self-interest to act contrary to his own self-interest, in an immediate situation, of course, not 'in the long run' [109]."

Physicians conform to their social role by placing the welfare of patients above their own—for example, by being available for emergencies or by reducing or omitting fees. In return, physicians generally receive respect, are addressed not as Mister, Miss, or Mrs. but as Doctor, and earn a higher average income than most professionals. In short, "to whom more is given, more is expected," a biblical aphorism frequently expressed by Dr. Albert Schweitzer.

"ONLY HE WHO IS A GOOD PERSON CAN BE A GOOD DOCTOR" (A. NOTTNAGEL)

The validity of this quote from the renowned nineteenth-century physician, Adolph Nottnagel, initially seems obvious; yet upon reflection, the "good person = good doctor" equation is simplistic. A kindly person should be a kindly doctor; yet that person might not be a competent doctor. Moral probity is not necessarily synonymous with job capability. In fact, in certain fields, such as politics, these attributes may be mutually exclusive. There are physicians, moreover, who are excellent professionally yet cheat on their income tax, and others who, though married, are indefatigable philanderers. Human beings can compartmentalize their behavior in the fulfillment of their different roles. Admittedly, physicians who are psychopathic or addicted to drugs and alcohol will be encumbered by their personal problems and may harm patients, but fortunately they comprise only a small minority of doctors.

Just as not every person is a born flight attendant, so not every individual is a doctor or a patient by nature. Through proper training and an effort to recognize and remedy deficiencies, most with at least average intelligence can become effective practitioners. So also can one learn to be a "good" patient—through the exigencies of the medical situation, proper instruction from the doctor, and appropriate support from family and friends. The role of the patient requires dependency, with which all adults, even those seemingly most independent, are familiar, primarily because they were all once infants and children.

But some patients have great difficulty acknowledging their dependency, which illness and disability intensify. For them, denying their deep desire to be cared for has been an important mechanism for achieving independence. The discerning physician should be alert to the basis for the behavior of those who "protest too much" about accepting patienthood.

How does the relationship between the patient and plastic surgeon begin?

Many years ago, at an annual meeting of the American Society of Plastic and Reconstructive Surgeons, I took a course with Dr. Gustave Aufricht, the doyen of rhinoplasty. His first words to us were: "Of course, to do a rhinoplasty properly, you must have a patient." To those of us starting a practice, his observation had painful cogency. I am now fortunate enough to have patients, but sometimes I am amused and surprised by the circuitous course of referral. In the United States, where we will allegedly have a surfeit of doctors in another decade, alternatives already exist for choosing a physician. Little has been written about the process of finding a physician under elective conditions. Until recently, when advertising, though still vulgar, became permissible, patients usually selected physicians through a personal recommendation: from family, friends, doctors, or nurses. Local and national medical societies probably account for a relatively small number of referrals. The yellow pages and newspapers with advertisements for cosmetic (rarely reconstructive) surgery are unfortunately becoming more important sources of information for patients. As these irregular channels to the plastic surgeon become busier, the path from the family physician becomes less traveled. An additional reason is that many patients do not have a family doctor.

While it is true that certain types of patients may gravitate to certain kinds of doctors, this phenomenon is probably less seen in plastic surgery than in other medical areas where the doctor-patient relationship is protracted: internal medicine, general practice, gynecology, or psychiatry. For many patients, their interaction with the plastic surgeon will be short-lived, and they might overlook a lack of empathy and sympathy by reasoning that "it will be over soon." Admittedly, this will be far from an ideal doctor-patient relationship but it might still be workable. Later if they should wish additional plastic surgery, they will probably find another doctor. With more plastic surgeons available now than even a few years ago, the patient at the outset does not need to feel constrained to accept an unsatisfactory situation.

The physician—specifically for our purposes, the plastic surgeon—chooses also his or her patients. This process may occur in various ways. Someone who does only esthetic operations will not see those who require reconstruction. Hand surgeons will not treat patients with head and neck tumors. High fees for consultation and operation may eliminate the relatively poor. Some plastic surgeons dislike "minor" procedures, such as excision of lesions, and these patients will either not receive an appointment or will be given one so far in advance that most will seek another doctor. Some surgeons and some patients do better with those of the opposite sex or with a different personality. One patient may feel secure with an authoritarian doctor, whom another might find arrogant. A surgeon's sense of humor might relax some patients but annoy others. From these observations, it is apparent that many factors influence the choice of doctor and of patient.

The Setting

Another variable of the initial consultation is the setting: a private office, a private clinic, a clinic at a teaching hospital, an emergency room, or the patient's bedside.

The patient who has an appointment with a private surgeon already knows at least the name, if not the reputation, of the physician who may perform the operative procedure. In many clinics, especially at a university hospital, the patient generally does not know beforehand who will be the surgeon. The reputation of the hospital or the medical school, not that of the individual surgeon, is what brings patients to the clinic. It does not necessarily mean that care here will be worse than it would be with a private doctor; in fact, it may be even better, but the settings and circumstances are different.

In the emergency room there is no elective aspect to the surgery. Frequently the patient is not sufficiently oriented to choose a surgeon or to discuss unhurriedly either details of the proposed surgery and its risks, or alternative methods of treatment. A hospitalized patient who is seen in consultation also has only limited options. The consultant is usually from the staff of that hospital. Opinions by physicians outside the pale are subtly or blatantly discouraged even though the patient might benefit.

Patients may fear that in a private office they will be exploited for financial reasons; in a university setting, they may fear they will be used for teaching purposes. Even in a private office they frequently ask, "Who is going to do the surgery?" The spectre of the "ghost surgeon" is strong. The patient's questions should be answered honestly and clearly.

One should remember that patients in the office are isolated from their usual environments. They are on your turf. If a member of the family accompanies the patient, you may gain some idea of the family dynamics but only at a distance and only partially. On a few occasions, I have made a house call, usually for a patient who has a decubitus ulcer and for whom a visit to the office or hospital would be a great inconvenience. One has then the opportunity to see patients in their own surroundings, among *their* pictures and photographs and interacting with *their* families. The doctor thus observes the patient in vivo in contrast in the in vitro office visit. Yet even in the home of the patient, we do not see him or her healthy and at work; thus our knowledge of the person is still partial.

YOU AND YOUR OFFICE
For purposes of this book, I have chosen to focus on the office, which is the most common setting for the first elective interaction between a plastic surgeon and a patient. During the time spent

waiting for you, the patient consciously and unconsciously has formed an impression of your office and you. In reality, you are your office. The way you furnish, decorate, equip, and manage your office is an extension of yourself. For this reason, every physician is or should be aware of the image he or she projects and wishes to project.

A plastic surgeon who wants to do only esthetic surgery, for example, is more likely to have as reading material *Vogue, Town and Country*, and *Cosmopolitan* than *Popular Mechanics, Scientific American*, and *Baseball Digest*. The intended slant is toward upper-class women who wish to maintain their beauty and not toward the factory worker with a hand injury or a basal cell carcinoma of the face. Whatever the reading material, keep it current. Patients resent out-of-date magazines that are crumpled and torn. Their displeasure is compounded if they see that the magazine is a discard from the doctor's home. They dislike being considered second best.

The way a doctor desires to be seen is frequently not the way others see him or her. Some patients in a lavish office may feel reassured and comfortable because the doctor seems to understand the rich and powerful and would appear also to be successful and wealthy. Other patients may regard fancy furnishings as a facade and as evidence of the doctor's penchant for expensive things obtained by charging excessively high fees. That patient may believe that the doctor, though presumably competent, is a poseur and is on the make professionally.

Qualities that patients universally appreciate are those that we like or should like most in ourselves: honesty, competence, concern [139]. Most patients expect their doctor's office to be clean, orderly, and attractive. Admittedly, decor differs with geography. What may appear modern in Beverly Hills might seem distastefully slick in Boston.

These considerations about furnishings are not minor since they affect the relationship between patient and plastic surgeon. How you may appear to the patient depends largely on how you think of yourself. Some plastic surgeons consider themselves plastic surgeons; some, as general surgeons with a special skill; some, simply as physicians; and fortunately, only a small minority as vendors. If the office and the demeanor of the doctor and the staff resemble more closely a beauty parlor than a medical facility, the patient will conclude that no "real operations" with real risk are being done here. Any complication will then be harder for the patient to accept because the stage has been set for a hazard-free medical jaunt. The ambience of the office may produce a more vivid set of expectations in the patient than any informed consent with its detailed disclaimers.

Your personal style should be evident, not a decorator's fashion grafted onto you like a poorly matched piece of skin—unless, of course, your style is somebody else's fashion. In the words of Yves Saint Laurent, "I like style—I don't like fashion. Fashion disappears. Style remains."

Anatomy and Physiology of the Initial Consultation

Let us consider the what and how of the first encounter between patient and plastic surgeon. Although the initial consultation may bring together two people who have never known each other before, the scene has been set long ago. Into that meeting, each carries an established personality with behavior patterns evolved from innumerable responses to countless stimuli; each has had thousands of social interactions—for the patient, some probably also of a medical nature. The doctor too has likely been a patient on more than one occasion, although one factor that limits the empathy of the physician is generally good health. The patient and the doctor will likely behave in a way that each perceives as the proper role for being the doctor or being the patient—roles culturally defined and passed from one generation to another. Were Hippocrates able to witness a consultation in a Boston office in 1980, he would see a ritual familiar to him although the dress and props would have changed.

In theory, the patient and the doctor could interact in infinite ways; in reality, they do not [10, 11, 15, 45]. What happens is remarkably circumscribed; perhaps there is unpredictable variation, but always on a predictable theme. This does not mean, however, that correct judgment is not necessary for both to take the wisest course for each.

The patient and the doctor are conscious to some degree, not totally, of the impression that each is creating; each is acting differently from how he or she would under other circumstances—for example, at a cocktail party or at lunch with a friend. The doctor-patient consultation could serve as an excellent illustration of what Goffman has called "the presentation of self in everyday life." He has written [53]:

When we allow that the individual projects a definition of the situation when he appears before others (a group or another person), we must also see that the others, however passive their role may seem to be, will themselves effectively project a definition of the situation by virtue of their response to the individual and by virtue of any lines of action they initiate to him. Ordinarily the definitions of the situation projected by the several different participants are sufficiently attuned to one another so that open contradiction will not occur. I do not mean that there will be the kind of consensus that arises when each individual present candidly expresses what he really feels and honestly agrees with the expressed feelings of the others present. This kind of harmony is an optimistic ideal and in any case not necessary for the smooth working of society. Rather, each participant is expected to suppress his immediate heartfelt feelings, conveying a view of the situation which he feels the others will be able to find at least temporarily acceptable. Maintenance of this surface of agreement, this veneer of consensus, is facilitated by each participant concealing his own wants behind statements which assert values to which everyone present feels obliged to give lip service . . . when an individual appears before others he will have many motives for trying to control the impression they receive of the situation.

This process of "impression management" and the awareness of self and the role(s) that each of us is to play has evolved to prevent or lessen social breakdown [136]. Within any stable society, most people do what is expected—drive on the correct side of the road, give a gift when appropriate and receive a "thank you" in return, go to the restroom labeled *Men* or *Women*, and so forth. In any given situation, no person exhibits his or her full potential. We neither say everything we think nor do everything we could. Accordingly, we never or rarely know someone else's every thought. We see only some of that person's actions, and our vision is influenced by what someone wants us to see as well as what we are predisposed to seeing. Under most circumstances of everyday life, these limitations do not impede the successful outcome of our transaction. For example, consider the instance of my going into a department store to purchase a tie. At the counter, as I am making my selection, I am aware of the salesperson, who is a young attractive woman (I have instantly noted her sex, race, age, physical attributes). I may even deduce from her rings whether she is married. Unconsciously or consciously I have already observed how she is dressed and how she is interacting with other customers— well spoken, efficient, pleasant? And she has surveyed me but most likely not with the same thoughts as mine. She will know, of course, my sex, race, and approximate age. She may judge my appearance less in terms of physical attractiveness than in terms of potential for buying: He looks well dressed and prosperous. These observations become even more important if her salary is based on what she sells. The chances, however, are that her income is fixed. Perhaps it is 4:00 in the afternoon. She is tired and bedraggled, yearning to leave the store after just one more hour. Inwardly, she may groan when I appear. Yet, mustering a smile she will invariably say, "May I help you, sir?" From the many possible replies, I will most probably say, "Yes, please." I have noted that she called me "sir" and I have had a fleeting twinge of disappointment with that further evidence of my aging—I may also wince because she is about the age of my daughter. None of this, however, ever gets expressed and she will probably never know my thoughts. (For her part, she may think "He is my father's age.")

The litany of our relationship continues—predictably:

SHE: Cash or credit?

I: Do you take Visa?

SHE: Yes.

While she is processing the sale and as she puts the tie into a bag, she may think, "What a dull tie!" But she would never say it. To break the monotony, I may offer something like, "The store seems really busy today" (certainly not a Churchillian phrase to be treasured by posterity). Mechanically, she will acknowledge it by mumbling, "Yes, it is." Or, to her surprise and mine, she might smile, look up and say, "You should have seen it yesterday. I was really strung out then." Tie in hand, I leave the store. I have learned nothing about her background (unless she has a distinctive accent), her life's dreams, her pleasures, or her pains. Nothing intimate has been exchanged. Any attempt in this direction would have been justifiably interpreted as forward, inappropriate, perhaps bizarre. Yet, an hour and a half later, that same person will be relating in a much different fashion to the man or woman in her life. Under those conditions, her thoughts and actions will differ from what they were in the store but they will follow a somewhat predictable pattern. For her boyfriend, who may pick her up at work (predictably at 5:15), a kiss (as soon as she gets into her seat she will lean to the left and he, to the right), perhaps a sigh more of relief than of passion, she will settle back and light a cigarette, glad that the working day is finished. He or she will ask "How was your day?" And so on, each reacting with the other according to expectations and experience. Only in a mental hospital, perhaps not even there, could the following sequence occur:

HE: How was your day?

SHE: Turnips are lousy to eat.

HE: Cronin is running for mayor.

SHE: (No response—keeping silent for an hour.)

She will not pick her nose in front of him nor will he drive on the left side of a two-way street (even in Boston).

The vignette of my purchasing a tie or the salesgirl with her boyfriend are mundane events in ordinary living. However, those happenings make up most of life. Let us now return to what might transpire at the time of the initial consultation.

The patient and the plastic surgeon will establish a relationship that has features common to any relationship between two human beings and between any patient and any doctor; yet it will also have aspects distinctive of the specialty of plastic surgery.

Recognition and communication characterize the process by which two people get to know each other. There is an exchange of information and feelings, largely through language and intonation; but what is not verbalized can be as important or more so than what is [33]. The body also communicates—by facial expression, gesture, and posture, for example. Within the first few minutes or even seconds of the initial consultation, the patient and the physician have appraised each other. In a computer fashion, each receives and stores information about appearance (attractive, neat, well dressed, or not), about manner (concerned, likeable, friendly, honest, or not), and about intelligence (bright or not). The patient will quickly form an impression of whether he or she can trust that doctor with the diagnosis and treatment of his or her problem. The physician also rapidly judges the patient, not only in terms of the diagnosis and possible treatment but also of the patient's capacity for cooperation. In what sequence and in what order of importance each evaluates the other is not generally known since it is complex and instantaneous; moreover, the assessment of the patient and physician will vary according to needs and values of the individuals involved.

Before meeting, the patient and the doctor usually know each other's gender. Undoubtedly, there are differences in the reactions of a doctor and patient according to the sex of the other. Though these dissimilarities in response may be subtle and momentary, they exist. Normally, the importance of the medical problem transcends or should transcend these considerations of sex. When there is ambiguity about gender, as with transsexuals, the physician, unaccustomed to these patients, may be visibly disturbed by not knowing how to classify them: whether to call them Ms. or Mr. or by what first name—and, in general, how to react to them [39].

Without venturing too far into the realm of psychoanalysis, one could safely postulate that the female patient will probably react to the physician who is male and older in some measure as she has related to other male authority figures: father, teacher, perhaps husband, and other doctors. Or she may sense the hostility of the male physician who has never liked women, perhaps because of an unsatisfying relationship with his mother or wife or both. Depending upon previous experiences as well as age differential, the male patient may view a doctor of the same sex as a grandfather, father, brother, son, or peer. I remember a male executive, about 10 years younger than I, immediately addressing me by my first name with the explanation that "I hope you won't mind. I always called my father by his first name."

Differences or similarities in race, religion, and socioeconomic status may also affect, at least initially, the interaction between patient and physician. In the United States, where we like to think that enlightened tolerance exists more than it really does, we avoid discussing these uncomfortable issues; but ability and need unfortunately are not the only criteria by which the patient and doctor judge one another. Each unconsciously and consciously holds stereotypes. Although this process may allow valid conclusions, it may also permit harmful prejudices. The patient and the physician may disregard important individual variations in formulating comfortable categories—"comfortable" because the familiar gets imposed on the new; each is navigating unknown waters. The advantage is ease; the disadvantage may be error.

The initial consultation does not arise de novo on a tabula rasa; the substrate has been present for a lifetime—two lifetimes.

Any action of a human being and any interaction with another can be broken down into component parts, small or large, and can be analyzed at different levels and from different perspectives: physiological, psychological (conscious or unconscious), personal, social, cultural, cross-cultural, religious, philosophical, cosmological.

Consider the geometric, stepwise description by the novelist Robbe-Grillet:

Then, holding the letter in one hand A . . . closes the drawer, moves toward the little work table (near the second window, against the partition separating the bedroom from the hallway) and sits down in front of the writing-case from which she removed a sheet of pale blue paper—similar to the first but blank. She unscrews the cap of her pen, then, after a glance to the right (which does not include the middle of the window-frame behind her), bends her head toward the writing-case in order to begin writing [121].

Tedious, mechanistic, yet accurate. Another writer with a different purpose and style might have stated simply, "she took some paper from the desk and wrote."

Similarly, the tableau of patient and doctor can be presented with broad strokes or in *pointillism*. My purpose is to make the reader aware that more is occurring than one might previously have believed, and that the tableau is not static but changing. The patient and the doctor meet for a short time in the continuum and complexity of their lives.

If one could analyze the patient's first visit in a time-frame sequence, it would become obvious that hundreds and even thousands of events take place. These happenings, moreover, involve numerous decisions, unconscious and conscious. For example, is the patient required upon arrival at your office to announce his or her name in front of the other patients? Where does your secretary (or nurse) tell the patient to wait, and where does he or she choose to sit? Is the waiting room for only your patients, or for those of doctors in the same specialty or in a different area of medicine? In this regard, one of my colleagues, who does esthetic as well as head and neck surgery (an unusual combination for these times), believes that those seeking cosmetic procedures will be repelled by the sight of patients who have had radical neck dissections, and therefore he sees each group on different days. Aside from the possible comfort of the cosmetic patients, he does not wish a prospective patient to wonder whether he who obviously does extensive ablation could also do or would be even interested in "delicate" esthetic operations.

A seemingly minor clerical procedure also involves complex decisions with various advantages, disadvantages, and consequences. Does one ask the occupation of the spouse? If so, who asks it, when, and why? Is it a means of reaching the family should an emergency arise? Is it to know the socioeconomic status of the patient in order to set the fee?

Other decisions concern how and by whom the past history and system review are obtained. Some doctors, like myself, view history taking as integral to the process of doctoring and they will use this occasion of securing information to help establish a relationship. Other physicians regard the history as a chore preferably done by someone else who, they feel, can do it as well as they, who are thus unencumbered to see more patients, increasing efficiency and income as well as decreasing tedium. Another alternative is to have patients make out their own questionnaires. Some patients resent doing this because they feel it is the doctor's job and not even that of the secretary or nurse. Advantages of having the patient do it include efficient use of time, a greater chance for completeness, and the fact that nobody knows the patient's past better than the patient. Furthermore, any information that is lacking or erroneous would be a result of the patient's error and not that of the surgeon or of anyone in the office. This possibly could be an important benefit from a medicolegal standpoint. Even though the secretary or nurse or someone else in the office may have access to information in the record, a patient usually has a greater sense of privacy if he is not made to divulge personal facts to someone who is not a physician. A major benefit of having the doctor or a trained interviewer obtain the history rather than having the patient supply it is the greater likelihood of being certain that the patient has understood the questions. Also, one can pursue a point if the answer seems significant. Responses to a questionnaire tend to be flat without clues to their possible import for the patient. The purpose of this discussion about history taking is not to champion one way over another but to illustrate that whatever course is taken, others are excluded.

The variations in taking a history and in running an office reflect the differing styles and objectives of doctors. Specifically, some plastic surgeons think of themselves as furnishing a service—an operative procedure—and view their interaction with the patient as a prologue and epilogue to what transpires in the operating room. Consciously and unconsciously, they do not want their relationship with the patient to be more involved than what is necessary to deliver their product. Perhaps they prefer distance in all their relationships. Other doctors, myself included, want more than a glancing encounter with a patient. I enjoy the depth and breadth of the more classic doctor-patient relationship. As a specialist, my surgical care is restricted to a relatively narrow-gauge track—but not so my concern for that person and his or her life beyond the problem that has brought about our meeting.

In addition to varying with the personality of the doctor, the routine of the office differs also with the locale: Standard office procedure in Juneau is not the same as in Manhattan. Moreover, the average type of doctor and patient in each of these cities is probably dissimilar, at least superficially in terms of life-styles, even though they may have the same ideals: peace, not war; kindness, not cruelty; longevity, not early death.

Since the patient has come to your office to get help, the reality is that the form and content of the initial consultation are determined more by your style and desires than those of the patient. Hopefully, your objectives will coincide with those of the patient but frequently this is not true. The physician who is overly aloof and insular may not perceive, much less fulfill, the emotional needs of the person in his or her care. Under these conditions, if the relationship proceeds to an operation, events unfortunate for both can happen.

FACE TO FACE

At some point you and the patient meet for the first time. After nearly two decades in practice and thousands of patients, I still find that moment exciting. Admittedly, I am less enthusiastic when I am tired or late or both. Yet even then I am conscious that this moment could be the start of a medical adventure or misadventure.

Your encounter with the patient involves several choices and decisions, largely on your part. Do you see the patient in an examining room, relatively bare, where the emphasis is on the physical aspects of his or her problem—the diagnosis and treatment? Or do you routinely begin in your office, usually larger than an examining room, and furnished in a style conducive to relaxation and to talking: rugs, pictures on the wall, mementos on the desk? In the former situation, your purpose is clear: no loitering allowed. You do not want to "waste time" with what you consider extraneous discussion or emotions. In the latter instance, you have provided more of a living room atmosphere and are trying to draw out the patient, to expand the boundaries of your mutual interaction.

How the patient arrives in the consultation area can also occur in more than one way. Is he or she led by the secretary or someone else who has called his or her name? Or does that person who is familiar with the patient from the preliminary paperwork preserve confidentiality in a crowded waiting room by a nod or a tap on the shoulder? Is the patient accompanied by someone or is he or she too afraid to ask whether you would allow this? Does the secretary or receptionist, knowing your desires, encourage or discourage a friend or family member to be present?

Once the patient is with you, how does the initial consultation proceed? Do you rise to greet the patient or are you already standing? Do you shake hands? Shaking hands establishes a physical contact, palpably bridging the gap.

Do you call the patient Mr., Ms., or Mrs., or by his or her first name? Do you call all children and most women by their first name? These matters involve more than manners. They are not inconsequential acts for many patients. For example, some older persons resent being called by their first names; some women reason correctly that they are being treated like children when they are first-named. Others, however, do not consider this form of salutation an act of disrespect; rather, they feel relaxed by the doctor's friendliness.

I remember a 70-year-old Boston banker who, while pruning trees one weekend at his New Hampshire home, cut his hand and, still dressed in his workclothes, saw "a young surgeon locally. He said to me, 'How did you do it, Billie?' Well, nobody but my father ever called me 'Billie.' I thought that that was as good a time as any to part company and I walked right out of his office."

Although the content and form of the initial consultation vary from doctor to doctor and according to the type and needs of patients [75], each doctor usually has a customary way of conducting the consultation. I am either standing or I rise when my secretary brings a patient in to see me—in my office (rugs, pictures, mementos). My secretary will say: "Mrs. Hodges, this is Dr. Goldwyn." I always shake hands and usually remark, "I am happy to see you." I then say, "Please sit down," and indicate a chair in front of my desk, behind which I then sit. A word about the seating arrangements: Next to the patient is another chair for a friend or family member. The desk, I recognize, is a barrier to communication. White [147] observed that when no desk intervened, about 55 percent of patients were "at ease," in contrast to 11 percent when there was a desk. I have consciously chosen to accept this impediment and to overcome it because I am more comfortable with structure that preserves distance while yet permitting friend-liness. Rightly or wrongly, I believe this is important, especially with female patients, who constitute about 75 percent of my practice.

I encourage all patients to bring in whoever may have accompanied them [59]. I will specifically ask the patient whether there is someone in the waiting room whom he or she would like to have present during this consultation. If there is, I sometimes ask either my secretary or the patient to go out to fetch that other person. Invariably, his or her presence will visibly relax the patient. By the time we are seated, I know whether or not the patient is somewhat relaxed or very anxious. Instead of jumping immediately into a new patient's problem, I will talk in general terms to relieve the apprehension as well as to get acquainted. "I see from the record that you are from Providence. I don't think that I have been there in a few years even though it is only an hour's drive away. How long have you lived there?" I might then ask what the patient or spouse does even though I have that information. Putting the patient at ease should be an early objective of the consultation. We must remember that a visit to the doctor is seldom a joyous occasion. Depending upon the problem, the patient may fear that his or her condition is serious, or that his or her desire for surgery will be considered "vain," or that your treatment will involve considerable pain, perhaps even death, certainly expense, and always uncertainty.

You should never assume why the patient is in your office. I usually begin with the question, "How can I help you?" I am conscious of using the word "can" rather than "may" because "can" implies an ability arising from training and skill. Other physicians might say "Why are you here?" or "What has brought you here?" or "What would you like to talk about?" If I know why the patient is here (from the record), I might say, "I understand you are here because you are considering facial surgery." Usually I refrain from that tack because it may either be incorrect or "too pushy." I am therefore aware of the impression I am creating by not looking like a huckster with regard to esthetic surgery. If, however, it is a noncosmetic situation, I may be more forward, justifying that approach by the fact that a cancer has instigated the visit. "I understand you have a lesion on your cheek. Dr. Wells told me that he just got back your biopsy report."

Never commit the grand gaffe of saying to a patient, "I guess you are here because you want something done about your nose," when, in reality, the patient is in your office because of a cyst on the back.

It is important to pay scrupulous attention to the precise words the patient uses in describing his or her problem. You will be able to learn the emotional reactions to it. For example, consider the differences in these statements of different patients:

"I have this thing [a nevus] growing on my nose and I can't stand to look at it." (Patient's concern is primarily appearance.)

"My wife is worried that this thing on my nose is growing. I had a sister who had a malignant freckle." (The patient's concern and that of his wife is melanoma. The patient has probably denied his fear for awhile and lets you know that he has made this appointment at his wife's insistence.)

"Dr. Smythe wants you to look at this on my nose. He thinks it's nothing but he wants to be sure. If it does not have to come off, I would be delighted." (The patient's concern is malignancy; the message is not to do unnecessary surgery.)

The usual progression of the consultation is toward the present illness. Here, as throughout your interaction with the patient, the focus can be narrow or broad. If, as I mentioned previously, you consider your role to be that of a vendor of a skilled service, you will not let your patients stray from the business at hand; you will want only the facts essential to determine fitness for surgery.

Aside from the realities of disease, we doctors, like everyone else, must contend with the reality of time. When the patient arranged the appointment, how much time was allotted? In some offices, the patient is asked over the phone the nature of the problem. While some patients might find this intrusive and annoying, it is necessary for the doctor's schedule as well as the patient's good. Generally, a patient with a small angioma on the cheek would require less time to see and to evaluate than would a patient desiring a complete facelift. Although some patients like the "in and out" approach, most do not. They may have waited many weeks to see you and, even if you consider their problem as minor—and it may be—they do not. In *The Thibaults*, by du Gard [36], the chief of medicine remarked: "The only thing patients really want is—to be taken seriously."

A patient with a small lesion may have a large medical history. Most physicians are clock conscious. This awareness of time is frequently communicated to the patient, who senses the doctor's impatience and may even apologize: "I am sorry to take up your time when I know you are so busy."

I have heard many doctors say, almost as a boast: "I need to spend just 10 minutes with a new patient." While it may be possible to effect an exchange of information, it is usually impossible to form anything more than the most tenuous connection with the patient if you give the impression that he or she does not really matter to you as a person but just as an object for an operative procedure. Admittedly, it is not only the quantity of time but the quality. Some physicians have the knack of being efficient without seeming pressed. Their manner is unhurried and the patient may feel that the time elapsed with the doctor has been at least half an hour when it has actually been only 15 minutes. However, there is for each patient an irreducible minimum below which he or she feels spurned and cast off. One of the most common complaints of patients is that "the doctor did not spend enough time with me." The patient usually does not mean that the doctor failed to diagnose properly or to recommend the correct treatment, but rather did not satisfy that person's emotional needs. Patients generally want to talk not only about their specific problems but also their fears, values, and their lives—what two friends would normally discuss with each other. The patient has entered your office as a stranger but wants to leave as a friend. Is that unreasonable?

The plastic surgeon who is not attuned to the numerous times in the course of the day that he or she has emotionally shortchanged his or her patients will remain oblivious to the well of dissatisfaction until something goes wrong; then comes the flood of hostility. But a broader and deeper relationship with the patient is not only useful to avoid later anger and unpleasantness but to give ongoing satisfaction to both the patient and the doctor.

In addition to the doctor's values concerning the profession, the consultation with the patient depends also upon the personalities of both. But because the doctor is in the driver's seat with respect to the fact that the patient has initiated the encounter, not vice versa, the doctor's preferences for the content and form of the initial consultation usually prevail. The more authoritarian the doctor, the more the consultation as well as the treatment are structured. Ideally, the doctor should listen more than talk. The purpose in asking a patient questions is to obtain information. Why interrupt the patient who is furnishing that information? The surgeon should not direct the consultation as if it were an operation. Letting it happen may have important dividends. Questioning, of course, is crucial to elicit relevant data and to channel the consultation within the realities of time. However, your queries should be gentle. You are a physician, not a precinct captain or a tobacco auctioneer. If, for example, a patient who seeks an augmentation mammoplasty is asked too soon about breast cancer in the family, she will become justifiably anxious and then will be incapable of listening and remembering what you have told her about the operation and its possible benefits and hazards.

The primary objective of the consultation for the doctor is to know the patient medically and emotionally. If there is to be a surgical journey, it starts then. Rushing the patient, scribbling down information with your head in your papers, and paying more attention to form than to content will prevent you from obtaining the perspective necessary for proper evaluation and treatment—the old "not seeing the forest for the trees" syndrome. The time that you take to sit back, observe, and listen will save you much more time and may spare you and the patient a serious error. The best occasion to know the patient is the initial visit. Someone once said: "All the major themes are present in the initial interview."

The consultation should glide and should not be a series of staccato acts. When it is time to "lay the hands" on the patient, it should not be done abruptly. If the patient's complaint concerns a usually unexposed part of the body, it would be best to take more time before examining him or her.

WHO IS PRESENT AT THE TIME OF EXAMINATION
Some physicians always examine the patient alone. My preference is to have a woman present (secretary or nurse) when seeing a

female patient for operative procedures of the breasts, buttocks, thighs, or genital area. Some patients request that only you be present; these patients usually have come for breast or chest surgery. They seem embarrassed by what they consider their deformity: small or large or asymmetric breasts, or a pectus excavatum.

Many times patients are accompanied by a family member or friend whom they want in the examining room. I do not consider this an infringement on my domain or the patient's, but rather an excellent opportunity to discuss the problem and possible treatment with the person who is probably the most important in the patient's life. That individual, moreover, will be able to recall the information that you gave the patient who is often so nervous about being there that he or she forgets what you have said. Also, an observer who is more dispassionate than either you or the patient might ask an important question that had not occurred to either of you.

There are occasions, however, when it is necessary to see and examine the patient alone. This is particularly true with a teenager inquiring about rhinoplasty. You may need information that the adolescent would be afraid to communicate with the parent present. Similarly, by separating husband and wife you may be able to find out more about their marriage to assess the impact of the procedure on each partner and their relationship.

Since patients differ, as do their problems, it is unwise to force everyone into a set sequence. Your system and style should have the flexibility of accommodating individual differences. The patient will then sense that he or she counts with you as a human being, not just another patient.

THE QUALITY OF EXAMINATION

The type of physical examination depends on the patient's problem: nasal deformity, parotid mass, mammary hypoplasia. How you examine is as important as what you examine. By that, I mean not only your competence but your gentleness and considerateness.

As physicians, we are so accustomed to inspecting, palpating, and probing the human body that we forget what it is like to be a patient. Since most plastic surgeons are male and since many patients for reconstructive surgery and most for esthetic are female, we must be aware of their feelings. In 10 or 20 minutes after having first met the patient, I may have learned about a problem that none or only few of her intimates know; I have listened to revelations about her personal life and her family history usually not discussed; and now, for example, I may be examining her breasts. What is routine for us physicians is certainly not for our patients. When I have my annual checkup, I am conscious of the embarrassment of standing undressed [125] before the doctor even though he is a friend of the same sex. Our society is still not unisexual in its attitudes and actions. Although most females accept the fact that most physicians are male, being nude or half-dressed in front of them is not without awkwardness and discomfort. Since I empathize with their situation, I usually say, "I know that most of us do not enjoy going to a doctor and being examined. I don't like it myself but I guess it is a reality that we all have to put up with." When I take their pictures, especially if they are of areas usually clothed, I say, "I know, Mrs. Burns, that you don't usually pose for such photographs." The acknowledgment of their ordeal with perhaps a trace of humor makes this part of the consultation more bearable for both the patient and myself.

I am never present when a patient of the opposite sex undresses since I believe that my being there will make her more ill at ease. Furthermore, how a patient disrobes is not relevant to the purposes of my examination, unlike that of a neurologist, who assesses the patient's ability to button and unbutton clothes.

THE PATIENT KNOWS
A common error of many physicians is to underestimate the intelligence of patients. This "intelligence" includes not only factual knowledge but perception as well. Most patients usually recognize hostility, hypocrisy, arrogance, avarice, and lack of sympathy, even when the physician thinks he or she has these traits well dissimulated. Someone, for example, who has been kept waiting inordinately will appreciate and recognize an apology that is sincere, not pro forma. If you are rushed, it is better to acknowledge that fact to the patient and perhaps suggest that he return (at no charge) for a proper, unharried consultation. Most patients will see through the pretensions of the room game, whereby, they are

moved from one place to another to give them the illusion that they are actually getting somewhere and that something is being done for them. As they go from room number 4 to number 1, the scene becomes reminiscent of an Arthur J. Rank production, with the gong expected to sound as the patient is finally brought into the presence of the doctor.

As much as possible, try to picture yourself as the patient. By so doing, you will soon find it easier to understand his or her emotions. That awareness will improve your patient rapport and your self-understanding.

No man values the best medicine if administered by a physician whose person he hates and despises.
JONATHAN SWIFT

BEHAVIOR BY THE PHYSICIAN OR STAFF THAT NEGATIVELY AFFECTS THE PATIENT.   Despite variations in personalities among patients and doctors and differences in office routines, certain actions by any physician, including the plastic surgeon, will be detrimental to the doctor-patient relationship [90–92]. Some I have mentioned already, but I wish to discuss them and others more fully now and later.

The pressures of a professional life can easily make us take for granted the patient's visit. We lose sight of the individuality of the patient; successive patients become a blurred parade. The physician may view the consultation as another chore; for the patient, this encounter with the surgeon is a singular occasion, a happening to be recounted to family and friends. Consider for a moment what the patient has gone through to arrive in your office. He or she has made an appointment, probably having made numerous inquiries concerning the "best" doctor able to take care of the problem. Most likely, the patient has had to wait a few days or weeks to see you and has had to arrange home and work schedules, probably also planning transportation and perhaps arranging for child care. A married patient's spouse may have had to take time from work in order to accompany him or her. The woman patient probably has thought carefully about what to wear for the consultation and has been worrying about what she will say, how she will respond, and what will be the course of her visit with you. If, indeed, her reason to be in your office concerns a major condition, such as an extensive neoplasm or a significant problem in esthetic surgery, she will be even more apprehensive. As physicians, we are so accustomed to dealing with patients who are anxious that we easily lose our empathy; we forget what trepidation is, unless that patient is ourself or a loved one [108].

Under these circumstances, the worst behavior on the part of the physician is an uncaring attitude [17]. The patient may make allowances for your being brusque, hurried, and harried, but will not excuse your lack of concern and sympathy. The patient does not want to feel like an intruder or a penitent. The most important patient is the one in front of you. Keeping someone waiting excessively (without apologizing), not listening, accepting telephone interruptions, signing or reading letters, and forgetting the patient's name are examples not only of bad manners but of inconsiderateness. They reflect your lack of esteem for that human being.

Writing about a house call Osler once made, a neighbor recalled: "In a room full of discordant elements, he entered and saw only his patient and his patient's greatest need, and instantly the atmosphere was charged with kindly vitality. Everyone felt that the situation was under control. . . . The moment Sir William gave you was yours . . . becoming wholly and entirely a part of the fabric of your life . . . he was one of those who having great possessions, gave all that he had [83]." In the office, the patient rightly views your staff as part of you. Passively or actively, a doctor thus condones the behavior of his or her helpers and associates. To patients, some secretaries are rude, unfeeling, and hostile. To overcome these liabilities, the doctor must labor hard to restore lines of communication. Frequently the patient is already angry before meeting the surgeon because of being treated so poorly when arranging the appointment and upon arrival in the office. Without realizing it, the doctor is already behind and must do more to get approval from that patient.

Detrimental to the patient–doctor relationship is lack of confidentiality. A patient whose name is called out in a crowded waiting room may feel embarrassed. Records carelessly left about so that names are easily visible may be noticed. Telephone conversations by the doctor or the secretaries may be audible. Some patients may hear friends being discussed and they correctly assume that they will suffer from the same lack of privacy.

Inefficiency of the physician and his or her office erodes the patient's confidence in the care that will be provided. The patient may surmise, correctly or incorrectly, that the doctor is not sufficiently interested in his or her problem to do what was promised. For example, the physician or secretary might have mislaid a letter from the referring physician, or the physician might forget to arrange laboratory tests or might not communicate the results to the patient.

Another point of irritation relates to finances. Pecuniary arrangements between physician and patient are admittedly important, but they should not dominate the relationship. Patients should understand their financial responsibilities, but should feel that the doctor considers their problem more important than their dollars. The surgeon who charges "excessively" in comparison to colleagues may be explicitly or implicitly saying to the patient: "I charge more but my results are better." If, indeed, the results are not so good as what the patient had anticipated, that doctor deserves the inevitable boomerang.

Obviously, improper diagnosis and treatment can shatter the bond between patient and surgeon. However, many patients can accept error if they have received kindness and truth.

It is regrettable that many physicians never learn the reactions of their patients to their behavior and that of the office staff. Physicians, like all authority figures, become insulated from the truth; they develop protective scotomata. Too often their reality is what is fed them by those in their hire. Part of the reason that it is harder to learn as one gets older is that fewer people dare to tell you your faults. Occasionally, the truth bursts forth from an angry patient but you may reject its validity as you are busy defending yourself from the onslaught.

APPRAISING THE PATIENT

To this fact, that we are each a secret to the other, we have to reconcile ourselves. To know one another cannot mean to know everything about

each other; it means to feel mutual affection and confidence, and to
believe in one another.
ALBERT SCHWEITZER
Memoirs of Childhood and Youth

After the physical examination, your interaction with the patient will concern his or her specific problem and your recommendations for treatment. In a later section, I shall discuss types of patients and types of operations; however, a word here would be relevant about what you have been doing thus far during the initial consultation. You have been assessing the patient in terms of a specific problem and that person's emotional and physical suitability for treatment, particularly operation. After half an hour or even less, and sometimes more, you and the patient will make a decision. In most instances, the judgment is correct although it is reached on the basis of incomplete evidence. No individual, even the physician with the greatest angle of vision, can see all facets of the patient. "A human life is always broader than we realize," observed Antoine, a physician in du Gard's *The Thibaults* [36]. Besides imperfect perception by one human being of another, there is also only partial comprehension of motivations. Blurred vision and faulty understanding are the givens of the human condition; yet despite these deficiencies, most of us adopt courses of action without fatal mishap.

Another point to consider is that even the most talented of us are biased by our very skills. We are prisoners of our own strengths as well as weaknesses. No matter how exalted we may sit, we are trapped on our perch. How different our species has appeared to Socrates, Voltaire, Marx, Freud, and Camus! Sometimes we physicians, in a supposedly rational occupation, forget that the patient in front of us still eludes the philosopher, theologian, political scientist, biologist, psychotherapist, novelist, and sociologist. We must also realize that we are connecting with that patient only briefly and at only one aspect of his or her being. The "care of the whole patient" is not only trite as an expression but is pretentious as an ideal. If such a holistic view goads us to be more understanding, competent, and compassionate, then it is worthwhile; but if it leads us to believe that we can truly fathom the entire patient and fulfill all his or her needs, then the concept nurtures arrogance.

The best that we doctors can hope for is to comprehend the patient well and long enough to help him or her, physically and emotionally.

Similarly, the patient will make a decision, perhaps more on the basis of trust than of knowledge. Ultimately, in every human interaction, there are no guarantees about outcome—marriage being an outstanding example.

A perfect relationship between a patient and a physician would bring together in harmony an ideal doctor and an ideal patient: a competent, caring, honest surgeon placing the patient's needs above his or her own, being always available, and charging well within the patient's ability to pay; and a patient with a significant problem for which there is a relatively simple solution, a trusting patient who will follow instructions with few complaints and few questions, someone who is grateful and will happily pay the bill.

Unfortunately, the world has few faultless people and consequently few perfect patients and surgeons. This does not mean, however, that most patients and most doctors will not have a satisfying interaction. The likelihood is that they will.

In this society to date, most patients are not assigned to a specific plastic surgeon, and most plastic surgeons need not accept each patient. In general, the more urgent the medical situation, the less important become the personality characteristics of the surgeon and the patient in their choice of each other. Whether a patient whose thumb needs replantation is hostile and neurotic will not influence the surgeon's decision to operate. However, if that same patient were there for an elective procedure, such as a musculo-cutaneous flap for osteomyelitis, the surgeon would do well to consider that patient's aggression before consenting to operate. Hostility in the individual who is in the office for a rhinoplasty would be or should be a reason to refuse to be that person's surgeon. In contrast to several decades ago when there were few plastic surgeons in the world, today's patient has more choice—as does the plastic surgeon, who need not feel guilty for refusing to operate if he or she believes the patient is a poor risk emotionally or medically or both. When and how to say "no" under what conditions will be discussed later.

2. Special Features of Plastic Surgery and Patient Selection for Esthetic Surgery

Although the range of operations in plastic surgery, both reconstructive and esthetic, is extensive, most procedures concern visible conditions of the skin, face, breasts, abdominal wall, and extremities. Results of surgery, therefore, are apparent and can usually be judged by patients and their friends.

The initial examination of the plastic surgical patient is regional and does not ordinarily encompass the entire body and, except for patients with a malignancy, it does not include vital organs, such as brain, heart, lungs, liver, or kidneys. A 40-year-old woman seeking a rhinoplasty, for example, would consider a breast or pelvic examination inappropriate if performed by the plastic surgeon; yet she would expect it in the office of her internist, family doctor, general surgeon, and gynecologist.

Except in the instance of trauma, most operations in plastic and reconstructive surgery are not emergencies. Even a patient with a head and neck cancer or a cutaneous neoplasm has the time to obtain a second opinion and to learn of alternatives of treatment such as irradiation or operation (and what type). Not so someone with appendicitis or an acute myocardial infarction.

Special Features of Esthetic Surgery: Confusion About Name and Definition

The first singular characteristic of esthetic surgery is the confusion about its name and definition as well as its spelling. Many plastic surgeons prefer the word *aesthetic* over the word *cosmetic,* wishing to avoid the connotations of makeup and a beauty parlor. The *a* that precedes *esthetic* in most communications from official organizations of surgeons doing this type of operation serves also to upgrade the image by conferring upon it a classic lineage. Since esthetic surgery is still fighting for rightful respect from the medical profession, even from many plastic surgeons who do mostly reconstructive work, another common practice is to use more impressive names for operations commonly called *facelift (rhytidec-tomy)* or *eyelidplasty (blepharoplasty), nose job* or *nasal surgery (rhinoplasty).* The invocation of Greek roots is indicative of the insecurity, frequently unconscious, among many cosmetic surgeons. In my presence, one head of a prestigious plastic service chastised a resident who listed the procedure as a facelift instead of a rhytidectomy, which the chief said would "look better to our colleagues."

Some surgeons favor calling cosmetic or (a)esthetic surgery the surgery of appearance or body-image surgery to imply more than the effecting of merely superficial changes. Pertinent are Gertrude Stein's comments: "A difference to be a difference must make a difference," and "Rose is a rose is a rose is a rose." The "official" definition of cosmetic surgery by the American Society of Plastic and Reconstructive Surgeons [3] is as follows:

Cosmetic surgery shall be defined as that surgery which is done to review or change the texture, configuration, or relationship with contiguous structures of any feature of the human body which would be considered by the average prudent observer to be within the broad range of "normal" and acceptable variation for age and ethnic origin, and in addition is performed for a condition which is judged by competent medical opinion to be without potential for jeopardy to physical or mental health.

Although unquestionably a courageous try at evolving an explanation helpful to insurance companies, therefore to patients and to surgeons, this definition is cumbersome. It demonstrates that occasionally it is easier to know what something is *not* than to define what it *is:* for example, beauty, love. The schoolteacher's maxim that "you don't know it unless you can define it" is not always valid. Furthermore, good reconstructive surgery almost always has also an esthetic objective [87, 122].

ENHANCEMENT

An important feature of esthetic surgery is that the patient considers the result of the operation an enhancement, not a loss as is usual after other types of surgery, such as cholecystectomy or hysterectomy. These benefits are objective as well as subjective. Because of an improved appearance, the patient becomes more socially desirable [93, 94]. Walster and associates [145] found physical attractiveness was the most important personal characteristic influencing how much one is liked in a man-woman dating situation. Especially for the woman, good looks are the passport to popularity and upward mobility. The confluence of beauty, wealth, and power is a universal phenomenon. Literally, it pays to be beautiful. Kalick [81] conducted an experiment in which subjects viewed preoperative and postoperative photographs. Individuals pictured postoperatively were judged to have more desirable personalities, to be better potential marriage partners, and to have happier lives than the same persons photographed before surgery. Since all the impressions were from photographs, actual personality was not a factor in his study. His findings and those of other researchers suggest that esthetic surgery may have a stronger social impact on patients' lives than had previously been assumed. The "enhancement" of appearance [52] from the operative procedure is not only in the mind of the patient but also in the minds of those around him or her. The improved social reception reinforces the patient's sense of well-being; glowing in these reverberations, the patient may become even more outgoing and charming.

The beneficial effects of esthetic surgery extend even to the patient's life at work, where advancement may be partially the result of an improved and younger look. Some executives, in fact, have credited their rise to a cosmetic procedure [89].

As plastic surgeons, we tend to be wary of the patient who wants an esthetic operation for job purposes. Our hesitancy is due to our fears that such patients will expect too much from the operation, and that if they fail to achieve their professional objective, they will be disappointed and even hostile. What we might consider unrealistic about the patient's expectations may actually be realistic.

ELECTIVE NATURE OF THE SURGERY
Unlike almost every other surgical situation, operating for esthetic reasons is completely elective, more so even than in other areas of plastic surgery. For the esthetic operative patient, survival is rarely the issue. Such a patient is usually in good health, which he or she is willing to risk in order to achieve a better self-image. The plastic

surgeon makes well patients ill in order to make them feel better—about themselves.

In esthetic surgery the patient who is least sick physically is in fact the best candidate. That individual fulfills least the classic sick role: The expected prognosis in terms of morbidity and mortality is excellent; anticipated pain is minimal; complicated ancillary procedures and prolonged nursing care are not needed. In contrast, the sicker the patient, the greater the likelihood that the operation is reconstructive, and the more the plastic surgeon, rather than the patient, becomes the judge of the result.

The fact that esthetic surgery is elective allows the patient and the surgeon time to decide. The patient can obtain additional consultations and frequently does.

GUILT AND EMBARRASSMENT. Esthetic surgical patients often feel guilty about wanting an operation that they, their family, or their friends consider "frivolous." They are ashamed about having an operation when they are not truly sick.

Although the popularity of esthetic surgery is increasing, the acceptance within the ethos of our Judeo-Christian heritage is still lagging. The Old and New Testaments speak against vanity and many patients coming for cosmetic surgery worry about being vain. An interesting contrast is that in the United States we admire more people who gain their money through work (achieved) rather than through inheritance (ascribed). In both instances, however, when people have either beauty from birth or wealth from their own work, the implication is that God has favored them.

Esthetic surgical patients are not the only ones embarrassed about their problem and their need for help [136]. Consider the person with a venereal disease or an emotional illness. In the former situation, society, while providing treatment, still is judgmental: "He should have known better." In the latter case, the often expressed message is that with enough will (ego strength), patients should be able to overcome their difficulties.

The patient for cosmetic surgery, especially if older, may receive little or no emotional buttressing from loved ones, unlike those persons with life-threatening disease, who are cajoled and sometimes carried to the doctor. Many esthetic surgical patients think that even the family doctor opposes the surgery they want. Their doing something of which friends and family disapprove increases guilt.

FINANCES.   For the cosmetic patient, going it alone as a *modus operandi* applies also to financial aspects. Insurance plans generally do not cover so-called luxury surgery, nor will they defray the expenses of treating its complications. Prepayment is customary for esthetic operations, unlike other areas of medicine except, perhaps, for orthodontia.

RAPID RECOVERY AND LITTLE REGRESSION

Since most esthetic operations can be done under local anesthesia (usually with intravenous supplementation), patients do not lose consciousness but are awake or drowsy. They maintain contact with the environment. Patients for cosmetic surgery not only want to resume their normal activities as soon as possible but are able to do so sooner than those undergoing more major procedures. For the cosmetic patient, there is little incentive for secondary gain by prolonging recovery. Less regression thus occurs; the esthetic patient does not break stride for long. Serious strains in the patient-doctor relationship may arise, in fact, if a complication delays the anticipated early return to normalcy.

MINIMIZING OF SURGICAL REALITY

In the relationship between the surgeon and the esthetic patient, there are features and pressures that lead each to minimize the surgical reality [32, 61, 135, 140]. The surgeon may tell the patient about risks but not in such a way that the patient is put off; the patient may screen out the information because he or she very much wants the operation. If the patient truly expected, for example, an ectropion or infection or blindness from an eyelidplasty, he or she would never have it done. The surgeon, by doing the procedure under local anesthesia on an ambulatory basis (especially if it is in the office) wittingly or unwittingly perpetuates the notion that this is not "real surgery," which usually involves general anesthesia and at least two days in the hospital, with the implication of a greater likelihood of serious complications as well as of a longer recuperative period.

Our culture fosters unrealistically high hopes. An apparent paradox in our society is the mixture of myth and science, of rationality and irrationality. Technological prowess has led us to expect that "all is possible." We are primed to anticipate more than we are likely to receive. It is hard not to become a victim of false hopes in a land where cigarette smokers are depicted as winning a pliant beauty, not a fatal cancer; where cosmetics, clothes, dyes, and esthetic surgery hide the natural state; where perfumes, sprays, and deodorants mask normal body odors; where the media stroke the fantasy zones; where the citizenry are told that they are "created equal" to have and become what they wish, as if mere desire could transform somebody ordinary into a Giotto, or a Garbo, or a Getty; where people believe that with more money it will soon be possible to conquer cancer, heart disease, and aging so that we shall live "happily ever after"; where politicians thrive by avoiding unpleasant truths and by promising the undeliverable. For a populace spurred to grasp the golden carrot in this world, it is not surprising that frustration, disappointment, and anger are likely to be high if medical treatment does not meet expectations. Something or someone must be to blame even with an informed consent signed by the patient. The attorney thus becomes the ombudsman, often for those who have unrealistic expectations and enormous self-entitlement. Even the concept that everyone has the right to sue and to anticipate recompense is not realistic, since obviously not all plaintiffs win.

The surgeon, not just the patient, may have fanciful expectations. It is always the next patient who may be the recipient of his or her first perfect operation. Perhaps the surgeon's practical sense has been muddled by articles and presentations that show only faultless outcomes. Ideally he or she will be more objective than the patient, but both are interacting as products of the same society.

PREPONDERANCE OF FEMALES
Another distinctive feature of esthetic surgery is that at least 90 percent of patients are females. The reasons are not anatomical, as in gynecology, but are cultural and personal. That most surgeons performing cosmetic surgery are men is also an important fact.

Our culture places a higher value on the attractive appearance of the woman than on that of the man; and the woman, deprived of the many sources of gratification available to the man, has learned to use and value her body, consciously and unconsciously, to please herself and others. This behavior is rewarded, perpetuated, and reinforced throughout her life by such acts as using makeup, adopting hair and clothing styles, and keeping "young and trim."

Inculcated with the desideratum of attractiveness and bombarded by measures and stratagems for acquiring it, many women feel obliged to change or maintain their bodies to promote pleasure for themselves and others. Aiding them in the battle for beauty is the plastic surgeon who, as noted, is generally a man and does not think it is unusual for a woman to enhance her appearance through surgery.

HAPPINESS AS AN OBJECTIVE

Esthetic surgery involves the elusive objective of "happiness." Results of psychotherapy are also judged in terms of that hard-to-define (and acquire) mental state; whereas in most of medicine, the efficacy of therapy is usually measured in decreased pain or increased motion or function (e.g., ability to defecate or urinate normally). It would be unusual to ask a patient after colectomy whether or not he or she is "happy" with the result. Being "alive and well" and "free of disease" are the common indices of success. The term *patient satisfaction* is rife in esthetic surgery but rare in neurosurgery or general surgery, for example.

Patient Selection for Esthetic Surgery: The Importance of Caution

Some patients should not have cosmetic surgery; their soma or psyche makes them unsuitable [5, 62, 115, 117, 118]. As plastic surgeons, we justifiably place great reliance on technique; but contrary to the message in most surgical atlases and sex manuals, technique is not everything. A well-executed procedure does not necessarily produce a happy patient. When one considers the vagaries of surgery and wound healing, as well as the complexities of human nature, it is surprising that so many patients seem satisfied with their results [52]. Let us consider identifying those who might prove to be the unhappy few.

THE PATIENT WHO WRITES AN EXCESSIVELY LONG LETTER
TO ARRANGE THE INITIAL CONSULTATION

The patient who thus approaches you is not simply providing information but is pleading his or her case. Generally, such letters contain an obsessively described saga of repeated dissatisfaction following multiple treatments of a condition that may be objectively less major than the patient believes. This compusive quality in recounting the excruciating litany of medical misfortunes is pathognomonic of a neurotic, rigid person who tries to relieve anxiety by attempting to control every item in life. Such individuals tend to be so perfectionistic that no result would ever please them (see pp. 42–43).

Now you will become the patient's last resort because of your "great reputation." The letter is not only an outpouring of grief but also a means of manipulation, to get you to don the armor of the knight errant for the patient's next surgical crusade. Almost always the patient will strongly criticize another plastic surgeon for lack of skill and sympathy. A common expression is "Now he won't see me or even return my call." Indeed, that might be so. Although this patient might appear pathetic and wronged, tread warily before deciding to operate, since you may well end up not as the knight errant but as the erring knight. Obtain all possible information from the patient, the family physician, and the other surgeon(s). Likely there has been more than one procedure by more than one surgeon.

THE RUDE OR "PUSHY" PATIENT

Some patients refuse to accept the next open appointment but insult or try to bypass the secretary to have you see them earlier. Frequently, a beleaguered referring doctor will apologetically call to have you see the patient as soon as you can just as "a personal favor." This type of patient wants to be treated as an exception because she (the patient is usually a woman) feels that she is exceptional. She has a high titer of self-entitlement that she will maintain until the last good-bye, which perhaps should be soon after the first hello. She will want the earliest possible date for surgery, a private room, and will insist that she be the first on your operating schedule. The "pushy" patient may later not accept your instructions and may become very hostile should even the slightest thing go awry. Usually these patients are well-to-do and may be accustomed to having all obstacles wither before their financial clout. As physicians, we should not discriminate against patients because of their economic status—poor or rich. Recall the interchange between Ernest Hemingway and F. Scott Fitzgerald, who observed: "The very rich are different from you and me." Hemingway replied, "Yes. They have more money."

THE UNKEMPT PATIENT

The unkempt patient is not out of place in an emergency room but is unusual in the setting for cosmetic surgery. While it is true that some patients with a pervasive deformity such as overly large breasts "let themselves go," a dirty or slovenly appearance may indicate a severely disturbed personality. Not every patient can afford a Calvin Klein dress, but all can purchase a bar of soap. With this type of patient, it is important to obtain an extensive medical history, including possible previous or current psychotherapy. Ask specifically about the abuse of drugs and alcohol.

THE PATIENT WHO MAKES YOUR OFFICE HER (OR HIS) HOME

Occasionally, you may find in your consultation room a patient who has taken over: looked through your papers and at the pictures on your desk, and taken books from the shelves. In my experience, these patients who aggressively rummage around your office are women. They wish to be in control by establishing an immediate intimacy. Some may ask whether they may be on a first-name basis with you. Their behavior may indicate underlying anxiety about dependency and perhaps they try to allay their disquiet by dominating every situation. This type of patient is trying to direct her own care. If you plan to operate upon her, you must establish early that you are in charge. To your surprise, they usually acquiesce very easily, almost thankful that you now carry the responsibility for them.

THE PATIENT WHO PRAISES YOU EXCESSIVELY AND
DENIGRATES YOUR COLLEAGUES

Some patients have discovered an eternal truth: Few can resist flattery. By plumping your ego, this type of individual may get you to do an operation whose result he or she will never like. You will soon join your confreres on the hate list.

The usual dialogue is like this:

SHE: I am glad you could see me. I've waited many weeks to come here. I'm thankful to be here. I've learned a lot about you. You certainly have some reputation!

YOU: (shifting uncomfortably in your chair): Thank you, but what can I do for you?

SHE: I am here to get your opinion and your help about my nose, which, I hate to say, has been butchered. I am sure you have heard of Dr._____; he is supposed to be good but twice he operated on me and my nose is worse now than it ever was before. My husband and friends don't know how I ever went through all I did—the pain and expense, and for what? A ruined nose? If he really thought he couldn't help me, the least he could have done was to tell me and refer me to someone like you.

And so it goes. The web is being spun.

THE PATIENT WHO GIVES A FALSE HISTORY

You may suspect an occasional patient of not telling the truth. Although apparently alert and intelligent, he or she may give contradictory information or seem surprisingly vague; dates may not jibe; the social and occupational history have an unconvincing, fictional quality.

I have had several patients who denied previous cosmetic surgery but had the stigmata of a rhinoplasty and the scars of a facelift. The patient may say that you are the first plastic surgeon she has seen but her questions and reactions to your replies belie her. One woman on whose lids I noted scars confessed when I questioned her, "I didn't want to tell you I had my eyes done a year ago. I wanted to see if you thought I needed surgery. If you didn't, I would have known that he did a good job." In that instance, fortunately, he had done "a good job."

Other patients may have an abnormal affect, as if they are sedated or tranquilized. Indeed, some are on psychotropic medication. They will try to hide their emotional illness, perhaps fearing that you might reject them for surgery. In this regard, they are not unrealistic.

If you believe that the patient has not been truthful, you should try to determine why—usually by gently confronting the patient with the inconsistencies of the history or physical findings or both. In general, with patients who act in this fashion, you are unlikely to establish a mutually satisfying relationship. Once the golden moment for trust has passed, it is seldom regained.

THE INDECISIVE OR VAGUE PATIENT

Sometimes a patient may be unable to tell you what bothers him or her. A woman may say that she is unhappy with her nose—her whole face—but, "What do you think, Doctor? Look me over and tell me."

This attitude characterizes a patient with poor self-esteem. It is best not to venture a harsh appraisal that would increase that person's dissatisfaction and expand the area of his or her surgical concern. The indecisive patient may schedule and reschedule surgery, to the exasperation of your secretary. Such vacillation is an indication of a lack of preparedness to undergo the operation and possibly even indecision as to what body feature really disturbs him or her. If you make the decision for the patient, he or she can then blame you for any later dissatisfaction, saying that you talked him or her into an operation.

A few years ago, a fellow surgeon consulted me for an eyelidplasty. On three occasions, he made arrangements and then canceled. Finally, I wrote him a letter (marked "personal"), in which I pointed out that his behavior suggested a conflict about having the operation or, at least, having me do it. I proposed that he seek another plastic surgeon. It was a hard letter to write because he was a doctor, but I fought against the temptation of treating him differently from any other patient. Later, he did have an eyelidplasty but was not pleased with the results, which to me looked satisfactory.

THE PATIENT WITH MINIMAL DEFORMITY

The worst combination for a satisfactory surgical result is the patient with maximal concern about a minimal deformity [98]. Since surgery is potentially hazardous, the object of the procedure should be of sufficient significance to warrant the risks. A patient whose emotional energies are directed toward a minute bump on the nose had better first see a psychiatrist. If, indeed, a rhinoplasty were performed, the focus of that person's dissatisfaction would then be on either the postoperative result or another part of the body.

I do not believe in tightrope surgery, in which you place the patient and yourself at hazard. If your operation is successful, what have you really done? If you fail, you have given the patient an unfavorable result, perhaps permanent, something truly worthy of anxiety.

THE PATIENT WHO REFUSES TO UNDRESS FOR PROPER EXAMINATION OR REFUSES TO BE PHOTOGRAPHED
Understandably, few people like to disrobe before a doctor or nurse, particularly if he or she is of the opposite sex. However, if a patient absolutely refuses to submit to a proper examination, then you cannot recommend proper treatment.

Many patients fear that their photographs will be used in a publication without their consent. They need specific reassurance about this.

Unwillingness on the part of the patient to be photographed may also prevent you from having an adequate record for planning. Furthermore, should medicolegal problems arise, your defense would be much weakened. The problem here is more than shyness. You should emphasize to the patient that you cannot proceed to help unless you can visually document the problem and thereby properly plan surgical treatment. Photographs to plastic surgeons are like blood sugars to a specialist in diabetes—this you might offer as a comparison. Help the patient to understand that your office routine has evolved from the care of many others with similar problems.

THE PERFECTIONISTIC PATIENT
We refer here to the individual who wants everything in life, including surgical results, to be "perfect"—every wrinkle gone or "the nose just so." It is usually impossible to satisfy that person because surgery and wound healing are beyond absolute precision

and control. The skin is not marble. Perfectionistic patients are hard on themselves and on others.

Instinctively, we plastic surgeons who tend to be perfectionistic can sympathize with anyone who seeks the faultless outcome. The combination, however, of a perfectionistic patient and plastic surgeon is frequently imperfection, so far as the result is concerned.

The perfectionistic patient frequently becomes the shopper.

THE SHOPPER

There are many very good people who are not what I call good patients. I was once requested to call on a lady suffering from nervous and other symptoms. It came out in the preliminary conversational skirmish, half medical, half social, that I was the twenty-sixth member of the faculty into whose arms, professionally speaking, she had successfully thrown herself. Not being a believer in such a rapid rotation of scientific crops, I gently deposited the burden, commending it to the care of number twenty-seven, and, him, whoever he might be, to the care of Heaven.
OLIVER WENDELL HOLMES
The Young Practitioner, in *Medical Essays*

The surgical shopper looks not usually for the lowest fee but for the surgeon who will guarantee the result. Like any shopper, this patient thinks of surgery as a commodity—something to purchase and to return if defective or if the buyer is dissatisfied. Unfortunately, most surgical results are never totally reversible. Do not be flattered that this patient has selected you from the six others already seen. The other five are the luckier.

THE PLASTI-SURGIHOLIC
This patient, usually a woman, is the seeker and bearer of multiple operations. She may proudly recite a list of famous plastic surgeons who have operated on her. Though relatively young, she may have already had her nose and eyelids done, her breasts augmented, and her abdomen tightened. She may want repeats or something new. That she has needed to submit her body to surgery and its attendant pain indicates her masochism and low self-esteem. This patient needs a psychiatrist, not a plastic surgeon, but

characteristically, she will refuse your referral and will continue her search for a willing surgeon.

It is easy to get trapped into operating on such a patient to correct a deformity, such as unsightly scars, resulting from her previous surgical escapades. You may delude yourself by thinking that you are not doing an operation but a "touch-up." Your remedial procedure still counts as surgery and it will be just one more notch on her belt.

THE ACQUIESCING PATIENT

Sometimes a patient wants an operation to please someone else, often to save a failing marriage. It is a form of masochism in which no surgeon should get involved. Willingness of someone to risk harm, to undergo pain, and to submit to another operation to improve an acceptable result from a previous procedure indicates psychopathology. It is a *folie à deux* for a surgeon to operate on this person without the benefit of psychotherapy.

Later, you may be surprised to see the husband and wife lovingly unite to blame you if the operation has not produced the desired result, anatomical or psychological.

A 55-year-old man, accompanied by his wife, came to see me because he wanted his nose made smaller and his chin larger. Significant in this history was a serious myocardial infarction two months before. In listening to his desires and seeing the marital interplay, it was obvious that his wife was the instigator. Her commitment to the surgery was strong and did not waver when I pointed out to her the risk of operating on someone so soon after a heart attack. I refused to do the surgery at that time and referred them both to their family physician, who at first seemed surprised that I doubted that this couple had a happy marriage. Later he called to say that after having talked with them further, he found out that the husband was impotent and his wife "could not stand him because of his big nose and small chin." Subsequently, they went for marital therapy for problems which, I am sure, were of greater importance than the size of his chin and nose. I have not since heard from them.

Another common instance of an abnormally compliant patient is the adolescent who accedes to rhinoplasty to placate an overbearing parent (see p. 77).

THE PARANOID OR DEPRESSED PATIENT

Elective surgery, especially if cosmetic, is best not performed on individuals who are paranoid or depressed [106]. With psychotherapy, that person perhaps may be prepared for operation, but its timing must be carefully chosen. The surgeon must communicate with the psychiatrist, whose clinical judgment hopefully will be sound. Occasionally, because of an impasse in therapy, a psychiatrist might refer a patient for plastic surgery—as a means of getting over the obstacle. Whatever the opinion of the psychiatrist, do not perform surgery if you have strong doubts. The patient may go into a reactive depression and you will have to bear the brunt of his or her dissatisfaction and anger.

Depression is not always obvious. Many seek plastic surgery after a loss, such as a divorce, a breakup with a lover, or the death of a loved one. Usually the patient is a middle-aged woman. The operation is desired to attain a younger appearance, almost as if the patient were trying to be born again—to start life anew. Often such patients could benefit anatomically from surgery, but it must be correctly timed to avoid further depression. Sometimes a consultation with a psychiatrist is helpful to be sure that the patient has experienced a proper grief reaction.

The loss and the subsequent depression need not always involve a person. The cause may be a change in financial status (down usually but up occasionally), or the loss of a body part, as for the mastectomy or hysterectomy (see p. 128).

A 43-year-old single woman sought a facelift for months after having had a hysterectomy and bilateral oophorectomy for enlarging fibroids. She was still angry at the gynecologist whom "I just can't talk to; he says I am babying myself." She thought that she had aged dramatically since her operation although, in fact, she had only the most minimal signs of aging, nothing sufficient to warrant a facelift. Listening to her, I noted that she was obviously depressed by what she considered her loss of youth, femininity, and fertility. She said that recently her spirits were better than when she had called for the appointment. At the end of the consultation, she seemed relieved to hear that many women under similar conditions have a depression and seek a facelift or other cosmetic surgery, from which they (herself included) would benefit very little.

Although there have been reports [37, 78] of success in performing esthetic surgery in patients with severe emotional problems, these happy outcomes should be considered feats and exceptions. The surgical blade is not a psychic knife.

THE PATIENT IN PSYCHOTHERAPY

The fact that a patient is in psychotherapy is not by itself a contraindication to esthetic surgery; it may be an advantage. It does mean, however, that you must ascertain the nature and degree of the emotional problem that led him or her to seek therapy. In addition to making observations, you must rely on the therapist for information about the patient. You must communicate with that therapist to be certain that what the patient seeks surgically is appropriate and realistic in relation to the ongoing psychotherapy, as well as to other aspects of the patient's life. It is surprising how often a patient who has been seeing a therapist for many months two to three times weekly has not discussed arranging a consultation with you. In these circumstances, as with any patient in psychotherapy, you should offer to call or write the therapist. A letter is preferable because your thoughts are then on record; also, it may elicit a letter in return, which will be part of the patient's file. Customarily, I dictate the letter in the presence of the patient and/or send the patient a copy, indicating to the therapist that the patient has either heard or will read my opinion. This openness helps to eliminate ambiguity and the patient's feeling that if surgery is refused, it was because of a collusion between the therapist and you. Frequently the patient will ask you to defer writing until he or she has discussed the consultation with the therapist.

For many patients, the undertaking of esthetic surgery represents progress toward resolving emotional problems and improving their life. Sometimes, it may be a hopeful shortcut around an obstacle in therapy. You must be very wary of that situation, since being in therapy can mean many things. The patient may be ready to terminate by agreement with the therapist or may be impulsively terminating without the therapist's approval. Or, the patient may be just beginning a difficult course in treatment.

Who the therapist is also makes a great difference. The task of treating emotional disease has been undertaken by many who are poorly trained and who are not psychiatrists, social workers, or clinical psychologists. Even within those groups are persons of poor judgment or meager experience. You may find yourself in the disquieting position of disagreeing with the therapist—almost always being more dubious than the therapist about the patient's ability to benefit psychologically from the operation. You may be forced to request an additional consultation, even to the point of suggesting someone else whose expertise you trust.

Sometimes a psychiatrist may refuse to give an opinion about the patient's suitability for surgery, perhaps responding to your request for guidance with the comments, "The decision is the patient's." Although not making decisions for the patient is a standard stance of many therapists and ultimately may be beneficial to the patient, it may be exasperating to you. Resist your impulse as a surgeon to resolve the ambiguity by action—by operating. Since the patient's condition is not urgent, you also can be and perhaps should be noncommittal. To the therapist and the patient, you may suggest postponing a decision and regrouping in a few months.

Personally, I would never operate on a patient whose therapist is opposed to the surgery. Frequently, I refuse even when the therapist is in favor if I sense trouble ahead. Remember that you still have a primary responsibility for the patient should he or she be dissatisfied after operation. Just as the psychotherapist can be wrong, so can you. I am sure that some patients whose surgery I would not do have gone to someone else and have had a satisfactory outcome, anatomically and emotionally.

THE MALE PATIENT

Although more males are seeking cosmetic surgery, the majority of patients for esthetic surgery (85 percent) still are female. From their findings, Jacobson and associates [78] concluded that male patients are more likely to be "psychologically ill" than their female counterparts. Frequently they have a "conscious desire to dissociate themselves from the undesirable traits of their fathers, and an unconscious desire to dissociate themselves from the primitive rage at the mother from whom the father failed to rescue them and for whom they have ambivalent feelings." These men are particularly sensitive to "any perceived threats to male effectiveness. The cosmetic complaint is a symbolic representation of and an alternative to more direct ways of dealing with these conflicts."

With cosmetic surgery becoming more popular among men, those who have it are now more likely to be emotionally stable than were male esthetic patients of two decades ago [141]. Today these patients may be doctors, lawyers, teachers, clergymen, politicians, executives, as well as those in the visual arts and in the media. However, one must be very wary of those men, especially if older, who want a cosmetic rhinoplasty in the absence of trauma or respiratory obstruction. They will have more psychological problems and postoperative dissatisfaction than those for facelift, eyelidplasty, hair transplantation, otoplasty, dermabrasion, abdominoplasty, scar revision, or correction of gynecomastia. I agree with others who have noted the basic problem of sexual identity in men who desire rhinoplasty. Such a patient may be confused emotionally and intellectually about how masculine or feminine he wants himself and his nose to be. This conflict has practical ramifications for the operation that we perform. The patient may be undecided about what characteristics he wants for his nose, as for example, how long or short it should be. Whatever the surgeon does to the nose, the essential psychological problem persists. This fact may account for the postoperative attitude of these patients, who easily become hostile and litigious.

In the man, the nose is the only projecting midline structure other than the penis, and through displacement, it may be the focus of sexual inadequacy. The nose contains erectile tissue similar to that of the genitalia and it responds to sexual excitement, menstruation, and pregnancy. In many cultures and at different times in history, the size of the nose was equated with the size of the penis, hence virility. A common punishment for adultery in India 3,000 years ago and in Germany in the Middle Ages was amputation of the nose. The patient may be in your office to seek this symbolic amputation.

THE "SPECIAL" PATIENT (VIP)
The danger with the "special" patient is that surgical judgment may defer to status. The patient may want you to treat him or her

differently from others because he or she is "important." Without your being asked, you may make medical decisions for the individual that you would not make for other patients. Departing from your routine increases the chance for error. Realistically, no doctor treats everybody the same since we must take into account a patient's personality, intelligence, and background. However, you should be treating primarily the patient's problem, not his or her socioeconomic position. Throughout our residency training, most of us saw errors of management that would not have arisen had the patient been poor and from the clinic, rather than rich and from a Cadillac.

THE PATIENT WHOM YOU DISLIKE

Fortunately, the disagreeable patient is infrequent. She or he is the type of person who, if presented with a dozen roses, would note only the thorns. Their bitterness about life, their insatiability, their hostility will focus on you and their postoperative result, no matter how technically acceptable it may be.

In an emergency situation or for a condition that threatens the patient's life, we must accept the difficult individual. However, for elective surgery, especially esthetic, there is no virtue to baring your neck to the guillotine. For taking care of that patient, you will receive not a medal but more likely a subpoena.

In general, never do an esthetic procedure on a patient who is hostile to you at the time of your initial meeting. Seldom will you be able to avoid becoming the target of more aggressive feelings. Furthermore, if the patient has diffuse aggression or if it is centered on some other surgeon, you will most likely become the next target.

Unlike psychiatrists—whose work is to deal with many unpleasant emotions, such as hostility—we, as plastic surgeons, do not need and should not wish to become therapists. Avoid the temptation to nurture your masochism or megalomania—to want to be an Osler or Freud (they did not operate on such patients!). Realize that at best a surgical procedure may only temporarily calm or defuse a hostile patient but, more often, it may be another stimulus to his or her punitive sentiments.

The situation is very different when the patient becomes hostile during the course of your treatment—postoperatively. Your responsibility is to find the cause and hopefully to resolve the problem (see pp. 168–176).

Another circumstance in which you confront an aggressive patient with whom you must deal responsibly is the instance of someone hospitalized who has become unhappy and angry (hostile in the hostel) because of failure in management or simply because of the length of confinement. The medical problem and the patient's reactions are identifiable and understandable—frustration, fear of never getting well, and loss of power. Weiss [146] has written,

A sick patient feels he no longer has control of his own destiny, for his role as an independent doer has suddenly been reversed and has become one of relative or complete dependence. Not only must he depend upon his physician, but upon those who previously depended upon him, his family. It is not surprising, therefore, to find the patient is equally hostile to family members as he is to the physician himself, demonstrating the global nature of this loss. He has figuratively become "impotent," and he sees the physician, his sole treater, as omnipotent. This precipitates with him to new sources of hostility—the first is a function of the newly-developed dependence and the second is a secondary manifestation of his rage at the physician when he discovers that his intense, immediate narcissistic needs cannot always be gratified.

The patient in the hospital or even one who has been discharged and for whom things are not going along smoothly is much different from the physically well patient seeking a facelift, for example, but who has a palpable anger toward life and you.

For some surgeons, the issue is not so much the patient they dislike but the operation they detest. The poor patient then becomes by association the recipient of the surgeon's irritability and displeasure. One plastic surgeon told me frankly that he found facelifts "boring" and he did them only because they were an easy way to make money.

Other surgeons do not like the kind of patient who might wish a certain operation. A colleague confessed that he thought "rich women" who sought cosmetic surgery were "vain, childish, and self-indulgent." His attitude was reminiscent of a line in one of John Cheever's short stories, "God preserve me from women who dress like *toreros* to go to the supermarket [24]." Fortunately, this surgeon had enough insight, if not to change his feelings, at least to avoid operating on these patients.

Rarely can one do well what one does not like doing.

THE PATIENT FROM AFAR

The out-of-town patient may present a problem not only in relation to cosmetic surgery, but reconstructive as well. Furthermore, distance is a matter of degree and the patient's and doctor's conception of it. For example, I have patients for whom a 40-mile drive into Boston is a fearsome ordeal, much worse than for other patients who may come from much greater distances. To some doctors with an international practice nothing is "afar." Yet, some general points deserve mentioning about the patient who is not from your backyard.

As a physician's reputation grows, so will the radius of referrals. Most surgeons feel their ego glow when patients come great distances to get their opinion and to use their skills. Despite the obvious advantages, there are, however, certain problems [2].

The first problem is that both the patient and the surgeon are under pressure of the moment to decide on a course of treatment. Frequently, the result is an impulsive decision that could have been avoided if the patient had lived nearby and could have returned for a second visit. Another problem is that communication with the referring physician or other consultants is not so facile and direct. Proper discussion with family members, such as parents or spouse, may have to be sacrificed for the sake of scheduling.

The fact that the patient has made the trip to your office alone and has decided to have the operation far from home may lead you as the surgeon to overestimate that individual's self-sufficiency and to underestimate his or her anxiety, fear, and loneliness. The patient then goes through the operation outside his customary orbit and ordinarily without the usual support systems. These realities become especially important should a complication occur, when the patient may become increasingly anxious about the separation from home and family. An unfavorable result will necessitate contending with mounting expenses, since the stay may have to be lengthened or additional treatment may have to be undertaken and this will entail more trips. The fact that the patient's family may have disapproved of the operation engenders even more guilt. In the event of a postoperative problem, it is essential that the family, the referring doctor, and anyone else close to the patient be kept informed about what went wrong in your plans for its management.

Every patient from afar who has had an operation must remain nearby long enough for proper observation and care. In addition to the physical realities of an operation, the patient needs emotional support to deal with the inevitable stress. Commonly, for example, after a facelift the patient will become depressed and will require periodic reassurance. The doctor must be there to answer questions, which are not so much to elicit information as to renew the patient's confidence. When the patient goes home, it is helpful to have him or her write or call regularly.

The postoperative patient returning home may also have difficulty in obtaining proper follow-up should it be necessary. She or he may have seen a plastic surgeon locally and then decided to go to you for the operation. It will be embarrassing to return to the home surgeon, who might also resent being asked to do the cleanup work. Even the patient who had not consulted another plastic surgeon may correctly dread his or her displeasure at being passed over for the original treatment and now being called in in an emergency. It is axiomatic that the patient should not have to arrange for follow-up care; you should do this in a telephone call or letter, preferably both, to smooth the way. Hopefully your colleague will not be hostile because the patient exercised the right of choice in his medical care.

Some patients want to have their surgery done out of town to avoid the embarrassment of having people know that they had a facelift, for example. That is understandable, although it is an unfortunate commentary on the state of human understanding. Others, however, have come to you because they did not know that they could obtain excellent treatment near where they live. To them, the appropriate advice is to have their operation at home. Their physical and emotional resources would be needlessly depleted by having you as their surgeon, particularly if staged procedures were necessary, as in reconstructing a breast.

With the patient from a distance, as with every patient, the surgeon's decision should be in the interest of the patient and not simply for personal gain.

WHEN, WHY, AND HOW TO SAY NO

For most physicians who have been trained to say yes to responsibility, it is sometimes difficult to say no. This inability to set limits accounts in large part for doctors working long days and, in general, overextending themselves. In addition, because of their personality as well as their training, doctors like challenges. Occasionally, however, they may fail to recognize the true challenge— not the patient's surgical problem but his or her psyche.

Under some circumstances, refusing to operate is relatively easy if the patient requires no surgery: someone who has come for a facelift but has only minimal signs of aging, for instance—or a patient whose problem is best managed by another specialty, such as dermatology. In the latter situation, the patient comprehends and appreciates your unwillingness to operate. Incidentally, I do not charge a patient who, for example, came for surgical excision of numerous seborrheic keratoses but whom I refer to a dermatologist for simple management with liquid nitrogen. I usually send a letter to that doctor. If the family physician originally made the referral, I generally suggest that he or she be consulted for the name of a dermatologist; thereby, I do not preempt that physician's prerogative.

Another situation in which saying no is unambiguous is when you do not feel competent to do the operation required by the patient's problem. None of us should be reluctant to admit that someone else may be better qualified. It would be unwise and unethical to attempt an operation that you do poorly or have done so rarely that the patient would be in jeopardy. In most areas of the country, there are plastic surgeons nearby who probably have the needed expertise. Remember the guideline: Treat the patient as you would want yourself or a member of your family to be treated. In fact, admitting your limitations will ultimately increase your stature in the estimation of the patient, his or her friends, and the referring doctor. Someone observed, "You make your living by operating and your reputation by not."

Another reason for refusing to be the surgeon is that the patient's health will not permit it. This judgment is made for elective procedures, usually cosmetic, and is reached in conjunction with the patient's family doctor or internist. The patient will understandably be disappointed and you must emphasize that your decision has been made not for your convenience but in his or her best interests. Spend more time with these patients so that they will not feel coldly rejected.

A more difficult situation is one in which the patient could benefit anatomically from surgery but because of his or her personality, you do not want to undertake it.

To the "perfectionistic" patient (see pp. 42–43) I usually say that "My skills are not such that I can give you what you want. I doubt whether anyone will guarantee that kind of result. Unfortunately, the state of plastic surgery is not at the point where you could be sure of getting specifically what you want. Perhaps, some other plastic surgeon might be able to do better for you." That technique allows you to withdraw without offending the patient, who has the option of going to someone else [46].

Much more difficult is refusing the patient whom you dislike (see pp. 49–50). As gently as possible, I usually say: "For some reason, you and I do not have the same vibrations. If I operated on you, I really believe that we would be on different wavelengths. You would be better off with someone else."

It would be foolish for you, the surgeon, and unfair to the patient to plow ahead when you have many negative feelings. The patient will perceive your hostility and will react aggressively. Far better for you both to disengage at the outset.

For a doctor, how *not* to say no is illustrated by what Oscar De La Renta allegedly replied to an obese woman who asked him why he did not make dresses for people built like her. He said, "I am a designer, not an upholsterer."

WHERE TO START AND WHERE TO STOP
This cryptic heading refers to a common clinical situation: A 45-year-old woman wants only a bilateral upper eyelidplasty but her lower lids also need doing. I am usually reluctant to widen the scope of surgery, particularly for a condition that consciously, at

least, does not bother the patient. She should understand that the lower lids, if left alone, might look worse by comparison once the upper lids have been improved. The risk, however, is that the patient will think you are talking her into more of an operation and, should there be a complication, she will be angry at what she now interprets as your insistence and at her capitulation.

The issue here is not simply a matter of esthetics or finances but of philosophy—yours and the patient's. In general, the concept of "while you are there" or "while I am here" can be dangerous. Stick surgically to what truly disturbs the patient. You should not assume the obligation of refashioning that individual. Admittedly, the face is a totality but it does not necessarily follow that operating on one aging feature inevitably necessitates including another.

"HAVE YOU EVER DONE THIS OPERATION BEFORE, DOCTOR?" This query, which may come from the patient or from family or friends, is easy to answer if you can honestly reply in the affirmative. If the contemplated procedure is relatively rare, then an answer of no will not diminish you. However, if you have not done the procedure but others in your community do it regularly, you may feel reluctant and embarrassed to admit that this would be your maiden voyage. (It would also be your patient's.) Obviously, you should reply frankly and refer the patient if it is best for him.

Informed Consent

For thirteen years, I taught my tongue not to tell a lie; for the next thirteen years I taught it to tell the truth.
THE KORESTER RABBI

Although the subject of informed consent itself deserves a book, certain general points need mentioning here; other aspects and specific examples will be discussed in association with individual operations (see Chap. 3).

Properly informing the patient about contemplated treatment is not only logical but essential, medically and legally. In the latter context, with respect to malpractice, doctors are accused usually either of negligence or of failure to inform adequately (or both). Not only must the surgeon inform fully and correctly but he or she must be able to document it.

There are various ways to inform [7]. One can inform without imparting information. Witness billboard advertisements for cigarettes. The hard sell is in massive letters; the part about "hazardous to health" can only be read by an eagle. It is easy to recite a litany of possible complications without highlighting the most important. The monotony of their presentation will obtund the patient's critical faculty. In order that the patient will not slip away, the surgeon, consciously or unconsciously, is following the letter of the law but certainly not the spirit of either law or medicine.

WRITTEN INFORMATION
For many years, 18 to be exact, I resisted giving patients reading material concerning a contemplated procedure. Although I recognized that such information would decrease ignorance, ambiguity, and anxiety, I was reluctant because I feared that unconsciously I would rely more and more on the handout to answer questions to allay fears and gradually less on the initial consultation and subsequent interaction with the patient. I also disliked (and still do) the fact that such booklets tend to be impersonal and lack the warmth that I believe is essential to the relationship between a physician and a patient. And leading the patient from the cold to the hearth is one of my primary professional objectives.

However, following the example of others (see Appendix), I have begun to give patients something to read after we have met and discussed the problem and possible treatment. I have yet to overcome my feeling that printed sheets are the quintessence of what Trevor has called "retailing information." Yet, on the balance, I believe that printed information educates the patient, particularly by making him or her remember some of the points discussed during the consultation. Its review is important since studies have shown that even when printed information, in addition to verbal, is given to well-educated patients, most remember less than 50 percent. In view of that depressing statistic, what sort of recall or sense of reality would an inadequately informed patient have?

Neither is it surprising that patients are least likely to forget things that they perceive to be the most important, especially if these things are mentioned first [45]. Any minister, teacher, or politician would recognize this verity.

Reading material for the patient is helpful in the event that you have inadvertently omitted a topic. The thoughtful patient will use the booklets as another opportunity to ponder the proposed procedure and to ask questions if he or she wishes clarification. Another advantage is that the surgeon can record having given written information to the patient, who can acknowledge that fact by signature. This may prove important from a medicolegal standpoint.

That this printed matter may find its way into beauty parlors where it may have been left by one of my patients makes me uneasy, since I am aware that some surgeons of "overweaning ambition" have resorted to this ploy.

Audiovisual aids, such as films about the operation (preferably with you as the surgeon dubbed in) help reinforce the message. Be careful, however, that not just the best results are depicted. Otherwise, you can be accused of implied guarantee, as would occur if you had shown a patient slides of your most favorable outcomes.

Availing yourself of a blackboard is also a good way to demonstrate what you want the patient to remember, but do so only if you can draw well; if not, the patient will conclude that you are as poor a surgeon as you are an artist.

Further information about cosmetic surgery is available free to patients in the form of telephone taped messages sponsored by Blue Cross and Blue Shield and various medical societies. In Massachusetts, for example, these recordings are excellent and can be heard by simply dialing a number. This can be done from your office or the patient's home. Obviously, before recommending such tapes, you should listen to them to be certain that they reinforce what you are trying to tell the patient. Although you can have the patient sign a statement that he or she has heard them, just as with written and verbal information, there is no guaranteeing that the patient has either understood or will remember.

CONSENT FORMS

Consent forms usually are remarkable for their complexity and obliquity [73]. Most patients regard them more as a means to protect the doctor legally than to inform them medically [23]. In the Appendix are a few examples of what I consider to be good consent forms. Some plastic surgeons have one form for every procedure; some have a specific form for each operation. Giving in detail the limitations of the procedure and its possible complications would seem ideal, but one must be wary of overwhelming the patient with facts and jargon. Some colleagues make the patient sign the bottom of an information sheet and each paragraph of a consent form in the space next to which is printed, "I have read this carefully. I understand this. I have no questions about this."

With every eyelidplasty, for example, I discuss the possibility of blindness and death. Hearing about these catastrophes rarely causes the patient to decide against surgery. The human being adapts by believing that such misfortune will happen only to somebody else.

The logical question is, when should the patient sign the consent form. It is more practical if it is done at the conclusion of the consultation in the presence of a witness—someone in your office or the patient's friend or family member. However, the patient may want and deserve more time to read through and cogitate about the consent form and, more importantly, about the procedure that he or she is planning to have. Taking a copy of the form home and discussing it with the family is better for many patients who are not calm or in their usual state of mind following the consultation because of the excitement and anxiety that it may have provoked. In my experience, many patients who go home with the consent form return it improperly witnessed, but this can be remedied and is probably better than having the patient sign something hastily and claim that he or she was "pressured into something that I did not really understand or want."

Like Sisyphus, condemned to push a heavy stone up the hill to let it roll down and then to begin again, the physician, with every patient, must inform honestly and clearly. If the patient gives up the idea of the operation or goes to another surgeon, you have lost very little. In fact, you may have spared yourself much trouble. If you are not operating on that patient, you will probably still be doing surgery but on someone else.

Even with verbal and written information, calls and questions continue. As one patient confessed, "You probably have mentioned it somewhere on what you gave me but I guess I'm calling more for psychological support." Her statement confirms the observation that when someone asks a question, the primary objective is not always to get information.

Finally we should remember that the patient, no matter how well informed, and the surgeon, no matter how skilled, must be content with a certain amount of irreducible ambiguity; something may go wrong. Fortunately, the unwanted event happens only infrequently. Yet, when it occurs, the fact that is is an uncommon circumstance does little to console the patient or the surgeon.

BEING UNDERSTOOD IS NO DISADVANTAGE

In the presence of the patient, Latin is the language.
MEDIEVAL MAXIM

The matter of informed consent emphasizes the need for adequate communication between every doctor and every patient. Communication between two people who have the ability to speak and to hear a common language theoretically should not be a problem. Unfortunately, the reality is different. Witness the many books and seminars on ways to improve communication. Consider also the innumerable psychotherapists working with clients on bettering their capacity to say what they mean to people important in their lives.

The first requisite to verbal understanding between two human beings is a mutual desire to communicate and to be understood—a comparatively recent development in medicine. For centuries, physicians exploited the mystique of their metier; they kept a veil between the patient and diagnosis and treatment. The rationale, conscious or unconscious, was that the ignorance of the patient worked to the benefit of the doctor. One might even evolve a law of medical dynamics: Respect for the doctor increases in proportion to the ignorance of the patient. The shaman knows the value in not telling all. However, unlike the physician in Western society, he has few scientifically proven measures at his command.

Not until the fifteenth century did a medical text appear in the vernacular rather than Greek or Latin, the language of the educated minority. Traditionally also the prescription was written in Latin and/or illegibly, accomplishing the same objective of bypassing the patient's comprehension. I recall witnessing as a resident the hospital's decision to label patient's medications upon discharge. Society and medicine had finally reached the point that allowed the patient to know. Patients do own their bodies and have a right to understand what is being done to them.

There are times, however, when failure in communication is due to the patient's not wishing to understand. These situations frequently occur in association with cancer or some other grim disease, but they may also happen with patients seeking esthetic surgery who may deny to themselves the possibility of postoperative complications (see pp. 35–36).

Johnson has commented on another aspect of "doctor talk [79]." "The doctor's 'we,' by the way, is of special interest. Medical pronouns are used in special ways that ensure that the doctor is never out alone on any limb. The referents are clearly vague. The statement 'we see a lot of that' designates him as a member of a knowledgeable elite, 'we doctors.' " This use or overuse of "we" occurs less often in an office than in a hospital, where the very complexity and the many support systems provide ready refuge and a tempting labyrinth for the badgered physician. Johnson is correct that often the physician does not wish to be "alone on any limb." We doctors should remember that the patients also do not want to be alone and, of course, being or becoming ill (having surgery) tends to isolate them.

It was Talleyrand who said, "Language was given man to hide the truth." While we might disagree with his cynicism and his explanation of the origin of the spoken word, the message is irrefutable: People lie. This fact is responsible for much of the chaos in personal lives and on an international scale—wars. Human beings have yet to evolve to the norm of saying what they mean and meaning what they say [18]. For example, just the other day I heard that the National Park Service was going to kill a large number of wild donkeys in the Grand Canyon—for conservation purposes. To avoid public outcry they termed their plan "direct reduction." This lack of forthrightness is obvious with many other euphemisms that we use. So also doctors and patients may talk near or around something unpleasant or bury it with words [16]. Such behavior augurs poorly for what should be a collaborative effort, not a dissonant interaction, with each knowingly misleading the other. This matter is not just a moral issue to be addressed at a symposium of doctors and theologians. It has practical relevance, as we have just noted in discussing informed consent (see pp. 55–59).

Fees

Every relationship between the patient and the physician must involve a consideration of some kind of payment to the doctor. This is true even if the payment is waived.

With few exceptions, most doctors that I know do not enjoy the process of securing recompense for their services. Perhaps this is a result of their having in their core the image of the unselfish, "dedicated" physician. When I went to medical school and where I trained in general surgery, physician's fees, like masturbation or other carnal practices, were not discussed. Only during my plastic surgical residency in Pittsburgh, Pennsylvania, was I allowed to see how an office functioned. I observed then that physicians of great competence and compassion actually got paid and that they did not reek of the marketplace. Someone once observed that it is fortunate that money exists. What else would we use for payment of services [21]? Think of how many chickens a patient desiring a facelift would have to bring to the office!

In the profuse discussions about the cost and distribution of medical care, surprisingly little attention has been directed to the question of what determines physicians' fees [60]. Despite complex "relative value" schemes sufficient to choke a computer, many inconsistencies, inequities, and absurdities remain.

Before getting lost in specific enigmas, let us first try to recognize a few guiding generalities. Physicians are paid according to the service performed without regard to outcome. A radical mastectomy, for example, has an associated monetary value, irrespective of morbidity, mortality, or cure. Perhaps the genesis of this *modus operandi* was the justifiable reluctance of the earliest physicians (and us today) to guarantee health and survival, which are not completely within the control of any human being. With or without a skilled doctor, disease and death eventually supervene.

Another feature often forgotten is that a third-party medical payment does not depend upon the skill with which the service is performed. A careless colectomy will bring the surgeon the same fee as one done with finesse—in fact, perhaps more as the surgeon has to treat the complications.

Physicians are paid differently for their time and treatment. A total gastrectomy garners a larger fee than a herniorrhaphy. Such variations are allegedly related to differences in the complexity of the procedure, the skill required, and the potential hazards. Less understandable are the fee discrepancies among disciplines. Is a cataract operation twice as difficult as a cholecystectomy? Is an hour of a surgeon's time intrinsically more valuable than that of a psychiatrist, pediatrician, or internist? Why is the diagnosis of hyperaldosteronism worth the same as that of the common cold? In most third-party payments, a patient visit is a patient visit, a consultation is a consultation. In surgery, Gertrude Steinism ends because an operation is not an operation is not an operation.

Differences in monetary recompense among surgical specialties are not due solely to the realities of supply and demand. Of importance are less tangible factors. Therapies requiring manual dexterity seem to earn more than cerebration alone. A doctor performing coronary bypass generally receives more than does a colleague managing a patient with a coronary occlusion. Yet, in both instances, the physician is directing his or her efforts toward the same objective; restoring the health of the patient. Is the monetary hierarchy in medicine related to a hierarchy of the body? Are the brain and heart king and queen and the large intestine and liver merely the knaves? It becomes a "mediphysical" riddle.

What about the fees charged by plastic surgeons for operations for appearance, such as rhinoplasty or facelift? Since these procedures are elective and are an enhancement rather than a necessity, one might argue that the usual standards for fees do not apply.

Although for many of these patients, "cosmetic" surgery is rehabilitative, some might question whether their cost should be more than that of a lifesaving operation. Few surgical acts are more lifesaving than a tracheostomy or drainage of an abscess. Should that have a higher fee than a vein stripping or a median neurorrhaphy?

The practice of medicine, like other activities of man, lacks apparent consistency. In all human affairs, paradoxes abound. Cultures vary in their values. A ballet dancer in Russia, for example, engenders the great excitement and top money that a professional football star does in the United States. And here, a rock 'n' roll singer will make far more money than any elected or appointed public official, including the president. Pecuniary reward, of course, is not the only measure of society's esteem. A Supreme Court justice gains a different kind of respect than does a speed car racer.

SETTING THE FEE

When I began practice 18 years ago, I had available a fee survey prepared by the Massachusetts Society of Plastic Surgery to give its members an idea of prevailing charges, their range, and their average. Because of the Federal Trade Commission's considering such documents contrary to the best interests of the consumer, this fee schedule and others throughout the country were abandoned. However, the young practitioner must still decide what to charge. The present method is to ask other physicians, generally older ones.

There are three alternatives: to charge less than the usual, the same as the usual, or more than the usual. The first might have the advantage of attracting more patients who believe that they will save money. It also has the disadvantage of convincing some that you are offering less. Charging the same as others has the benefit of allowing the young surgeon to blend with peers. Charging more has the advantage of possibly making you more money and perhaps convincing some patients that your higher charges reflect your better care and skills.

Ultimately, the decision as to what to charge is determined by the attitudes and values of the physician as well as the means of the patient. The former is more important than the latter, although in many instances it should not be. The surgeon (or physician) must feel comfortable about what he or she is exacting for services rendered. Each of us must find a fee that is neither demeaning to us nor excessive to the patient. Of course, the possibility of establishing a fee exists more in esthetic procedures than in reconstructive ones, where third-party payment regulates the remuneration and may preclude additional charges.

There are some surgeons who charge so much that they are pariahs of the medical profession and have paradoxically earned a bad reputation for which they would willingly pay a public relations firm to untarnish. They would have been wiser to curb their materialism in favor of earning a good name. The cycle becomes inexorable. They soon suffer the disrespect of their colleagues and, as they become more ostracized, they take revenge or satisfaction in charging even more. They get caught in the "the more you make, the more you spend" trap. They are unhappy with less and require more. Their life-style becomes intensely demanding: They work harder, charge more, make more, and may be enjoying it less.

How another person conducts his or her life is not the issue here. But how a physician wishes to live and to charge to live that way does affect his or her relationship to patients.

Another aspect of fees deserves mention: the practice of some to charge excessively as a deterrent to the patient. I have heard colleagues say, for example, that they "cannot stand to do facelifts." Therefore, they set their fees so high that patients wishing that operation will be discouraged. The obvious question is why these doctors do not tell patients that they prefer not to perform a specific procedure. The reason is that an admission of a deficit in their repertoire would seem a weakness and such a confession, as they would interpret it, damages their self-image. They would like the patient to feel that he or she is inadequate financially, but not that they are surgically. The irony is that patients undeterred by the high fee will be paying a premium for the procedure at which the surgeon is perhaps least proficient.

Since very few physicians enjoy discussing fees with patients, many resolve the conflict by delegating that matter to someone else in the office. This tactic undoubtedly increases their income since patients are less likely to persuade someone other than the doctor to reduce the fee; in fact, they are less likely to ask. I confess that I still discuss my fees with my patients and still do not enjoy the process. However, there are instances when I believe that a lowering of the fee is justified and it would not happen if I were not a participant in the discussion. I realize that what I have just written might be an argument for the doctor absenting himself from this part of the initial consultation.

PREPAYMENT

Most plastic surgeons and most patients desiring cosmetic surgery expect prepayment. Since insurance does not usually cover these procedures, the patient must pay his or her own way—be-forehand. But this practice arose because of other factors besides the lack of third-party payment.

Empirically, collecting before esthetic surgery, rather than after, is easier. If patients postoperatively fail to honor the bill, the surgeon has only two alternatives: to forget it and be consoled that he or she has helped someone and probably also learned something; or to engage in unpleasant encounters with the patient and the court.

You cannot take back a performed eyelidplasty as you could a refrigerator that is unpaid for. Many surgeons believe patients are happier with their result if they have already purchased it. They complain less about scars, swelling, or residual wrinkles.

Basic, however, to the issue of prepayment is the fact that many cosmetic procedures fail to give the patient what he or she had expected. In my experience, this is particularly true of facelifts. A year or even six months later, a few patients look more pre- than postoperative. Not everyone comes out as well as those on the slides at meetings and in the photographs in books. And even if you technically achieve a surgical nirvana, a few will still be dissatisfied. In retrospect, because of their unrealistic hopes, they should have been weeded out during the initial consultation.

Aside from the patient and surgeon, prepayment has affected the emotions of our non–plastic surgical colleagues. Many are angry and envious since they perceive this practice as evidence of the easy materialism of our specialty. Explaining the reasons for this financial arrangement sometimes increases their understanding but seldom eliminates their negative feelings.

Near my home is a well-known restaurant where one pays for the meal beforehand. Although the food is good, this monetary routine leaves a bad taste. I can empathize with those who resent not just the expense but the idea that they are not to be trusted. Since other restaurants serve the same fare, I can go elsewhere, but a patient desiring cosmetic surgery has little alternative because prepayment is standard in the United States.

For perspective, it is interesting to realize that in the time of Hippocrates, physicians were accustomed to being paid before they rendered their care. When a doctor took on a patient, a certain fee was agreed upon for the entire treatment. The physician was not paid for every service. Hippocrates and his disciples, however, advised the doctor not to be "too greedy" and "to take the economic status of his patient into consideration, even to be prepared to give free services occasionally, either because he has some obligation toward an individual or for the sake of his reputation. This is especially desirable in the case of some poor foreigner who has fallen ill far away from home, without the possibility of obtaining the funds necessary for treatment [133]." The doctor was urged not to raise the question of fees in the beginning with patients suffering from acute diseases, since worrying about finances would worsen their health. Like many other precepts of Hippocrates, this still has validity.

PROFESSIONAL COURTESY
The term *professional courtesy* refers to the traditional reduction in charges to certain people, primarily physicians and their family;

however, other patients commonly receive this special consideration, such as nurses, medical students, residents, and clergy. Great
is the variation, both among doctors and geographically, in the
interpretation of professional courtesy [41]. In my practice, for
noncosmetic surgery, I accept third-party coverage as complete
payment. If the patient has none, I generally make no charge
either for consultation or surgery. For cosmetic procedures, I do
not charge doctors at my hospital with whom I have a close
relationship—nor their family, nor residents and medical students
and their spouses. With nurses, clergy, and with doctors whom I
do not know, I reduce my fee. For dentists and veterinarians, I
charge the usual.

The financial aspects of professional courtesy sometimes are not
so important as other, more subtle considerations. For example, a
colleague, who is a friend, may bring his wife to me not only
because he may like me and trust my work but because he knows
that I will not charge him the full fee or I will markedly reduce it.
His wife might be embarrassed by going to me because I know her
and her family. Later, should a complication occur, she will probably not directly express her anger for fear of creating a disagreeable scene in front of me, a family friend, or for fear of seeming
ungrateful after I have performed her operation for nothing.

The treatment of fellow physicians and their families takes place
in the hazardous zone along with any other VIPs, who are im-
periled by being treated more for who they are socially than for
what they have medically. All of us can recall with anguish instances when we changed the rules and the routine to oblige a
colleague or friend—with unfortunate consequences for all concerned. Professional courtesy, then, may still be for some a gra-
cious act; an exception that should affect the ledger and not the
therapy. That this ideal is not always possible to achieve is another
reason to abandon this practice, which financially squeezes the
doctor who may have many colleagues and their families as patients. My impression is that professional courtesy has become an
anachronism [8] although I am still struggling with it. Dr. Thomas
D. Rees has a tastefully printed card that is given to those patients
who might expect professional courtesy. It reads as follows [116]:

During the many years that I have been in the practice of Plastic Surgery, I have extended courtesy fees to close friends and doctors as a matter of principle. As the years pass, I have been fortunate in accumulating more friends and enjoyed the professional confidence of families, to the extent that almost one-half of my time these days is consumed performing such surgery. With the increasing costs of overhead in the practice of surgery today, not the least of which is our excessive and growing insurance premium for malpractice insurance, it is no longer possible for me to fully extend such courtesies. Needless to say, it is embarrassing and distasteful for me to have to charge my usual fees to close friends and colleagues; however, the practicality of the matter dictates that I do so. I hope you will understand and forgive me, since all I have to offer is whatever expertise I may have developed and my time.

Scheduling for Surgery: When and Where

Numerous methods exist for scheduling patients for surgery. In some offices it is done while the patient is there, immediately after consultation. Other surgeons communicate later with the patient. For some patients, calling or writing at a future time is more convenient because they do not have their appointment books with them and they usually have to arrange for time off or a babysitter.

Every plastic surgeon has personal preference as well as the reality of available beds and operating room time. Most patients want their surgery as soon as possible after they have decided upon it. Under some circumstances, either because of the patient's schedule or the surgeon's, the date may be months away. The long interval between consultation and operation may cause the patient uneasiness. I have found it helpful to encourage the person who wishes another visit to return a month or so before operation. Aside from reassurance for the patient, this occasion allows you a second look, to rethink your plans and to understand better that patient's personality and expectations. You will be surprised and disheartened by questions that you thought you had answered in detail before. You will then realize the wisdom of what Baptist preachers have long known: Repetition improves retention.

For you and your office, scheduling is a routine; for your patient, it is a singular life event, ambivalently contemplated: the pleasant hope of improvement coupled with the disquieting fear of failure.

Several doctors and a few patients have told me that it is unwise to fit someone into your operating schedule with the explanation that "someone canceled." The patient may then imagine that you are not good enough to hold that other person and he or she got away, off to someone better. The patient may then follow that example, real or imagined.

Frequently two patients will have consultations on the same day and will ask to be scheduled for surgery, also on the same day. In my experience, these patient duos generally are a mother and daughter for rhinoplasty or two women friends for facelift. They may even request the same room. Their plan seems reasonable and easy, but be careful because one is certain to do better than the other in terms of pain, ecchymosis, swelling, and final result, including scars. Even if both results are objectively very good, one patient is likely to envy the other (she probably did before the operation), and since she cannot rationally direct her hostility toward her friend or family member, you are the logical target. Tactically, also, whom do you do first on that same day? One is bound to feel slighted.

I require every patient on whom I do an operation to sign an authorization form (see Appendix). I cannot claim that mine is superior to others but it has the guarded blessings of several attorneys specializing in medicolegal matters. In truth, it does seem to have been written to protect me as much as the patient.

Because I do not perform surgery in my office, I discuss scheduling in terms of a hospital setting. Like any institution, hospitals are cumbersome to deal with. For the esthetic surgical patient, especially as an inpatient, care in the hospital is more expensive and less efficient than in an office operating room. Doing your surgery in your office has other advantages: saving time for you and the patient; preserving anonymity for the patient; facilitating uniform, presumably higher grade, medical care; and providing a relaxed atmosphere for the patient as well as you and your staff [113]. This is not the place and it is not my purpose to discuss fiscal benefits and liabilities or management problems of an office surgical unit, since others have written about these aspects [113, 127].

Pertinent, however, is the fact that within a hospital, you and the patient have the advantage of better backup of personnel and facilities in the event of a cardiorespiratory emergency. As the proprietor of an office surgical facility, your legal responsibility is greater, especially if you do not have a board-certified anesthesiologist in attendance. Another aspect to consider but not to belabor here is the progressive professional isolation of those who do office surgery from their colleagues and trainees not in plastic surgery. I am assuming that plastic surgical residents would be rotating through your office, although not every full-time chief sees the wisdom for this exposure. As the office-based, office-operating plastic surgeon becomes further separated from the main channels of medical care, the good that plastic surgery can do for other fields in medicine and surgery and for those patients diminishes. Likewise, the opportunities available to plastic surgery for germination decrease. These thoughts are expressed not to oppose office surgery, which I approve if high standards of patient care are maintained.

The trend is back toward doing esthetic surgery in one's own bivouac as was the practice in the early twentieth century. The rising costs of hospitals, the unavailability of bed space and operating room time, and the too-often flexible priorities of a hospital usually work against the esthetic surgical patient and his surgeon.

Another disadvantage of being a patient staying in a hospital is the possible confusion and mismanagement that can occur because of the large size of the institution, its inherent complexity, and the many people who participate in furnishing care. Unless nurses and residents are used to dealing with a cosmetic patient, he or she may be the target of hostility. ("With all we have to do, we have to look after someone like her who is healthy." "I hate people who have nothing to do but to get their face lifted."—a remark made about a patient who worked long hours as a legal secretary.) Envy may be the basis of the aggression ("I wish I was rich enough to do that. She even gets a private room."). There is a low threshold to considering a facelift patient as "demanding." One nurse made this judgment when a patient asked her five hours after operation for a glass of water because she had difficulty in doing it herself with the ice compresses on her eyes.

The surgeon who has hospitalized patients must be a fence

mender, taking the time to listen to complaints, minor to major, justified or not. While maintaining allegiance to his or her patient, the surgeon must hear both sides and not reflexively champion the person who is paying for the services. Most unpleasant incidents in the hospital readily resolve themselves with the realization that they probably arose because the patient was anxious and the staff member overworked. As the patient's physician and as someone known to those who run the hospital, your presence should be the constancy amidst the flux. Your availability and concern will reassure the patient and the participants in his treatment. For example, if you do not make rounds on a Sunday, call the patient and nurse to inquire about progress or problems. Most hospital rooms now have phones; certainly each nursing station does. Speaking with the patient requires a willingness and only a three-minute effort on your part, but the patient and the staff will greatly appreciate it.

In another context, after outpatient surgery, there is truth to what AT&T claims about the phone—that it is "the next best thing to being there." For a patient who has had a somewhat extensive procedure on an ambulatory basis, such as an augmentation mammoplasty, hearing from you the next day will be gratifying and helpful. Even with instruction sheets, there will likely be questions. The patient, however, will value your caring (if you do care) even more than your information.

Of course, doing these things requires you to be around. Avoid becoming "the will-o'-the-wispish surgeon"—now you see him, now you don't. Unlike the average physician of 75 years ago, today's doctors are not homebodies. The automobile and the airplane as well as the second home have made quick getaways a routine life-style for many. Leaving for the weekend or junketing to meetings is commonplace. Where does that leave the patient? Behind, and often angry. Even though you may have provided competent coverage, your surrogate is not the same as yourself. If possible, you should introduce the doctor covering for you to the patient if they do not already know each other. This is not simply good manners but good medicine; it cements your confrere's responsibility and lessens your patient's anxiety over being placed under the care of "only a name."

Particularly after esthetic surgery, it is best to be in town not only to handle complications but to manage depression. Your presence may mean even more than your words. If you have to go away on a trip and you know about it well in advance, you should not continue to operate up to the moment that the cab arrives at the door. Unfortunately, the economic realities as well as the demands of patients may make this advice more ideal than practical. At least inform the patient when you schedule him or her that you will not be there during the immediate postoperative period. Often the patient will choose to postpone surgery until you return.

Admittedly, doctors like anyone else need a respite. There are some patients, however, who require your availability as much as you do your vacation. They do not want to feel deserted. Proper patient selection and scheduling can usually accommodate both of you satisfactorily.

Who Should Know?

Sometimes it is difficult to decide whether to discuss the patient's problem and visit with anybody else: a family member, another physician, or a friend of the patient.

Take the least ambiguous instance first: Any plastic surgeon would consider mandatory revealing the content of a consultation with a parent(s) or guardian if the patient is a 14-year-old girl who had been seen alone or had been accompanied by a schoolmate. Because of her age, it is legally required in most states to obtain (parental) consent for operation.

But what about an 18-year-old girl who wishes a breast reduction but does not want the family to know about it since "they would only worry and they would be against it anyway"? Under these circumstances, my tack is to try to convince the patient that communication with her parents, for example, seems logical and fair. With proper understanding and knowledge, I venture, they might even support her plan. Usually, I say to the patient, if she is still opposed to telling her parents, that I feel ill at ease at "being in the middle," especially if something went wrong. If there were a complication, she would then have to tell them but under more stressful conditions. Most of the time the patient consents, but not always. I must then decide whether I am willing to proceed with that extra burden. The enormous geographical mobility of our population has fragmented the family; children and parents often lead separate lives and sometimes we are asking a patient to communicate when lines have long been down.

The fervor, success, and validity of the women's rights movement have made wives less dependent upon the approval of their husbands for their decision about an operation. The law does not require that a wife or a husband inform the spouse. The law also does not require that a plastic surgeon perform a procedure under these circumstances. Some of my colleagues will not operate unless a spouse sanctions the surgery. I require that he or she know that it is being done and give at least grudging assent. Also, I like to speak to the spouse about the contemplated operation but will not demand this if the patient says that the husband or wife is "violently against it." I try, however, to understand the basis of the spouse's objection and to offer them both the opportunity to speak with me about it. Sometimes, a husband may be opposed because of his fear that his wife will be harmed and will experience unnecessary pain. Also possible is the situation in which the husband does not want his wife to improve her lot because he is pleased with their relationship in which she, with her feelings of inadequacy, allows him the ascendant role. No surgeon likes the unpleasantness of being caught in the cross fire. Ideally, any operation is a family matter and it is better to have the husband and wife, together with the surgeon, all pulling in the same direction.

THE REFERRING DOCTOR
My custom is to send a letter to the referring doctor after I have seen the patient. Always, I inform the patient of my intention, since some occasionally will object, because, she (almost always a female) will say, "I asked him if he knew of a good plastic surgeon but I did not tell him that it was for me or what the problem was." Usually, in these circumstances, the patient has come for a breast augmentation, an eyelidplasty, or a facelift. Frequently the referring doctor is a neighbor from whom the patient obliquely extracted your name. The patient would not want him, particularly his wife, to know that she has had cosmetic surgery.

The End of the Initial Consultation

As with the beginning, there is an art to ending the initial consultation. It should terminate naturally, not abruptly by your unexpectedly standing up and saying, "Well, I think we've covered everything." The use of "we" is offensive and may not be warranted since the patient may still have questions and concerns. One who is even moderately perceptive will sense it when the skein has run out: when the patient and you truly have nothing more to ask or say. I always accompany the patient to the door, open it, and usually remark, "I enjoyed meeting you (if I did enjoy it) and I look forward to helping you (if that is true)." Often, before scheduling the operation, I prefer to let the patient think more about the contemplated procedure and to discuss it with family and friends, since now the patient presumably has more information than before the consultation. He or she may ask, "How do I schedule surgery if I decide on it?" My reply is, "Just call my office and speak with my secretary (whom I again introduce to the patient)." I also offer to answer more questions that might arise. If the spouse is not present, I state my willingness to communicate with him or her, either in person or by phone. Seldom does that happen. For the spouse, perhaps, the feeling of not being excluded by your having offered the opportunity to talk is more important than the information that he or she might receive.

On a few occasions, when I have spent a long time with a patient who has unending lists of questions, I have had to say, "Please forgive me, Mrs._____ (it is always a woman), but I am afraid that I am keeping others waiting. If you think that you would like another consultation, we can arrange it." Rarely is my suggestion accepted. Some physicians charge for a repeat consultation; I usually do not.

Occasionally a patient's final query will be, "Could I speak to someone who has had this operation (generally breast reduction or reconstruction)?" I try to discourage this, primarily because I believe that the patient ends up talking to someone who is pleased with the surgery—hardly an unbiased sample. Only someone who is happy with a surgical result would offer to converse with a prospective candidate. I point this out to the patient, but if she persists I then tell her that my secretary will try to arrange it, since we have a list of those who have expressed a willingness to do this. In order to preserve confidentiality, only first names are used. The patient is told to call at a certain time (set by the former patient) and to ask for "Mary," who has been informed that a "Janice" will be telephoning.

Just as I like to show a patient a range of results as, for example, with breast reconstruction, I wish I could have the patient speak to those who have had a poor outcome. But that is impractical because neither the patient nor I may relish further communication.

3. Types of Operations and Types of Patients

In this chapter, which is a discussion of specific operations, I have resisted the temptation to include more procedures than I regularly perform. The gain in completeness would be offset by a loss in authenticity. All surgeons, myself included, have a basic defect, perhaps congenital, that predisposes them to believe that they have performed a greater number and variety of operations than the facts allow. Like it or not, this is the era of the "incompleat" surgeon.

First I characterize cosmetic operations along with the patients who seek them. Subsequently I discuss reconstructive procedures. To generalize is admittedly a hazardous necessity. Casting someone new in the context of previous experience may be inaccurate, yet it is a proven mechanism for survival.

Rhinoplasty
THE ADOLESCENT GIRL

Most patients for rhinoplasty are adolescent girls. Generally, the patient has initiated the idea of modifying the shape of her nose but occasionally the mother, less often the father, is the instigator. The mother might have had the procedure or might have wanted it but did not perhaps because of financial reasons, parental unwillingness, or her own anxiety about the result. Most girls do not say they want a beautiful nose; rather, they wish to get rid of an "ugly" nose. They want to blend with their peers and not stand out because of an unattractive feature. Usually, the father is the last to concur with his child's wishes since he may see "nothing wrong with her nose" or his daughter in general.

How one teenager coped with her father's disapproval of a rhinoplasty is worth citing. She wrote him this letter:

Dear Dad,

I'd like to get your approval before I get a nose job so please try to see my point of view.

Getting my nose fixed is very important to me. I try to improve myself by going to school, reading, playing the piano . . . this is just another way that I can better myself. I think it's important that you allow me to change what it is I don't like about myself, because it would make me a much happier person.

I'm asking you to be totally unselfish and approve of something I want for the sake of my ego. I'm asking you to cater to my wishes and allow me to improve my appearance—which means so much to me. You've always been receptive to my needs, though, so I don't think I'm asking for too much.

Please think about this carefully, and try to understand how important it is to me.

Thanks.

Love,
Ann

In addition to discussions with her, Ann's father responded also with a letter:

Dearest Ann,

The measure of a person is composed of many things. These include the character of an individual, how one responds to internal and external events—the maturity one has, the intelligence, the accomplishments, how interesting one is. In all of these ways you are tops and Mother and I are very proud of you because of this. You are very intelligent, you are an excellent pianist, you read and learn so that you are very interesting. Your mind is always active and seeking to do other things such as gardening, weaving, etc. And on top of all this, you are energetic and physically attractive. It is because of these characteristics and your marvelous personality that you are so very popular and sought after by all.

You are also very pretty and have an excellent figure. This is fortunate because physical attractiveness is important to anyone's ego. But beauty of this type is very much an individual matter which has as much to do with fantasy as with anything else. Consequently, this physical beauty is very much a secondary characteristic that is totally unrelated to and very unimportant when compared to matters of character and achievements such as those you possess. Beauty is *not* an accomplishment.

This is difficult to understand when you are in your teens, an age when so much emphasis is placed on physical perfection. But it is important to try to understand so that now and, in the future, you become comfortable with yourself. Such comfort derives from the realization that each person looks different from another. Not only are noses different but hands, feet, other aspects of the face differ. It is just this variation that makes life so interesting. If you do not fully appreciate this and become comfortable with it, then restructuring your nose will be of no consequence—in fact, it will make your discomfort about other physical matters worse. If you do understand this, then restructuring your nose or any other part of your body would be unnecessary.

If your nose were so grotesque or so misshapen as to be obviously abnormal, I would not hesitate to agree with you. Fortunately, such is not even close to this situation. Never for one minute have I ever taken notice of your nose or thought that it looked unusual. I would suggest that you think about this matter for some time. If after a few years you still feel that it should be done, then perhaps this will be a correct choice.

Ann, I love you very much and I want to give you everything that I can and to feel that it is justified. One of those things is any guidance and insight that I might possess. I hope you believe and understand that.

Love,
Dad

What is obvious from these letters are the love and respect each has for the other. The father was correct about his daughter: She was attractive and accomplished. However, she was still unhappy about her nose, a fact which her father was somewhat slow or reluctant to realize. Ultimately, he did not insist that she wait "a few years" but after more discussion and a visit with me, he approved of the surgery and was warmly supportive.

A word about the age for operation. In general, I prefer to wait until the patient is at least 14, although there are exceptions, depending upon physical development such as age of menarche and degree of breast enlargement. Sometimes, harried parents will call to ask you what to tell their 12- or 13-year-old daughter who is pestering them for a rhinoplasty. In that situation, it may be helpful to see the young patient, who will follow your advice to wait whereas she will not heed it if it comes from her parents.

During the initial consultation it is important to establish whether the patient herself desires the rhinoplasty. As mentioned, she might be there because of parental prodding. A good opportunity for ascertaining the extent of pressure from her parents is during the physical examination, which logically allows you to be alone with the patient.

HISTORY.   In addition to a thorough past history and systems review, you must inquire about possible nasal trauma and breathing difficulties. The latter is frequently hard to establish because the patient may have been schooled by the parents to complain of that symptom to obtain insurance coverage. Later, your physical examination should clarify the situation. It is not uncommon for parents to attribute mistakenly, but honestly, their child's nasal deformity, such as a dorsal hump, to trauma and not to heredity. This thinking serves two purposes: It absolves the parents of guilt from transmitting to their offspring a displeasing physical feature; it also makes the surgery "necessary" for reasons of restoration not for those of vanity, which has been traditionally condemned by our culture.

Be certain that you question the patient and her parents about allergies (especially to medications and antibiotics) and bleeding tendencies, personal and familial. Before focusing on the nose, try to know that patient as a human being: What does she think of herself? What are her relations to her family and peers? Does she like school? How did she spend her last summer? What are her favorite subjects, extracurricular activities, and future plans? What does she think this operation will do for her at this time in her life, emotionally and socially?

PHYSICAL EXAMINATION.   On physical examination, it is important to ask the patient how she would like the nose changed. Occasionally what she wants is anatomically impossible. Better to establish that before you operate than afterward. Although you should examine the patient alone, it is helpful later to call in the mother and father to explain your evaluation of their daughter's nose and your surgical plans, and to determine the parents' expectations.

Dr. John Williams has emphasized the value of being gentle during your examination [150]. The patient is usually apprehensive and, as he has observed, may worry that you will find something "dirty" in the nose, such as normal mucus or crusts. If the surgeon forcibly grasps the nose, she may justifiably deduce that his surgical hand will be just as heavy.

Carefully inspect the complete extent of the nasal passages (with an otoscope or a speculum and headlight); note the presence or absence of septal or turbinate obstruction. Do not neglect to assess the patient's nose in relation to her entire face: forehead, lips, dental occlusion, and chin.

INFORMING THE PATIENT. As mentioned, the patient and the family must understand your surgical objectives. This is possible only if you understand them. Examine now and think later is a poor modus operandi. Though I refrain from showing pictures of other patients who have had a rhinoplasty, I believe a patient is entitled to know your operating plans since she must display your handiwork for the rest of her life. It is helpful to take a Polaroid picture (Polaroid SX-70 Land Camera, Abpha S.E.);* you can then immediately discuss the shape of the nose as it now is, as well as your contemplated modifications. A thorough discussion during the initial consultation usually obviates seeing the patient and the family for another preoperative consultation. A second visit, however, might be necessary if you, the patient, and family wish it, usually because of lingering uncertainty about your surgical objectives and their expectations. This additional visit is advisable for those for whom you can do less than what they wish, as in the instance of the patient with a bulbous, thick-skinned nose without a dorsal hump but with acne. If you plan external incisions (along the rim or at the alar base), inform the patient and the family about the expected scars.

I emphasize to the patient that rhinoplasty is not like sculpting marble. Human flesh is different and healing is unpredictable. Furthermore, one cannot throw away a nose as you would a piece of wood or stone if the result is unsatisfactory. Because the operation involves changing the foundation of the nose, its bone and cartilage, you and the patient must rely upon the soft tissues to contract to produce the final result. At operation, it is almost impossible to know precisely how the nose will ultimately mold and heal. Adding to the problem of knowing the final shape of the nose is the swelling from the local anesthesia and surgical trauma as well as individual variations in the shape of the cartilage, thickness of the skin, and its intrinsic ability to heal.

I outline the sequence and details of the procedure and the hospitalization. I do not do this operation, except for minor modifications or revisions, on an outpatient basis. I discuss the pain that the

*Polaroid Corporation, 784 Memorial Drive, Cambridge, Mass. 02138.

patient may expect (usually little), the type of anesthesia (local with intravenous medication), the length of the operation, the nasal splint worn for a week after operation, the expected time for discharge (usually the day after), and the fact that the initial swelling and ecchymosis will largely disappear in two weeks but many months will have to elapse before the nose assumes its ultimate configuration. The patient must be warned to avoid sports and other strenuous activities for three weeks after operation.

COMPLICATIONS.   The patient and family must clearly understand that complications might arise. I state openly that it is possible to die from the operation but it would be a rare event and, at least at this writing, I have not had a fatality from a rhinoplasty. Infection is uncommon, but unexpected nasal bleeding does occur in approximately one percent of cases (my series), although it is almost always controllable. Also I tell the patient and the family that in approximately five percent of cases it is necessary to do a minor revision, such as a minimal rasping of the dorsum, to achieve the wanted result. If septal work is necessary, warn about the possibility of perforation.

Many patients have misconceptions about the operation and postoperative regimen. For example, a common myth is that they can never again expose their nose to sunlight. Furthermore, some patients believe you can produce the type of nose they wish according to the picture they bring. They must understand the reality is quite different. I have refused many patients because either they or a strategic family member (usually the mother) expected too much and was so perfectionistic that she would make the daughter ultimately dissatisfied with her nose even if the outcome was very satisfactory.

DURING OPERATION.   Since most nasal surgery is done under local anesthesia with the patient awake, it is axiomatic that she should not be aware of unnecessary noise and careless talk: for example, "Whoops!"; "Even if her nose comes out fine, do you think it will help her because she is overweight?"; "The nose still doesn't look straight."

Another precaution is to send to the pathologist all tissue that is removed. A colleague and I reported a patient in whom we were doing a secondary rhinoplasty for a deformity partly caused by an unsuspected adenoid cystic carcinoma, diagnosed from the tissue removed at our operation [67].

Should the patient feel inordinate pain or have excessive bleeding, remember that it is not her fault. Too often I have seen surgeons become angry at the patient instead of directing their energies to rectifying the situation.

AFTER OPERATION.   Since rhinoplasty is the first of the operations to be discussed in detail in this book, I will emphasize something here that I need not repeat but feel is axiomatic for every operation: As soon as the patient is in the recovery room, you, not your secretary or resident, should communicate with the key family member or friend. The apogee of callousness is for a surgeon not to call immediately or to see and inform an anxious husband or wife, for example, about the condition of the patient, about the findings at operation, and what was done. Instead, too frequently a surgeon will dictate the operative notes, smoke a cigarette, have coffee, kibitz with colleagues, and then go to lunch. Someone so unresponsive in this situation to the emotional needs of others will probably be lacking in other contexts. The surgeon who believes that he or she is too big to perform this minor act of common decency is really too selfish. Anyone, the surgeon included, would be irate at not receiving a call about his own daughter.

When the patient after rhinoplasty is to be discharged, do not forget to speak to the family or whoever will be looking after the patient. Talking with you allows them to ask questions and, perhaps even more important, it gives them a sense of completeness and security. This type of communication demands little from you but adds much to your rapport with the patient and those important in his or her life.

Returning to rhinoplasty, it is fortunate that almost every adolescent girl will be happy with the result of her rhinoplasty [76]. This patient ignores flaws that might bother her family and her surgeon. Sometimes I feel guilty because the patient is ecstatic with a result that is far from faultless. I should add that I resist the temptation to point out the shortcomings.

If the parents or a relative or friend of great importance to the patient does not provide emotional support, even a good result might seem bad. In general, cosmetic surgery is a family affair.

THE OLDER WOMAN

The older woman usually does not want a significant change in the appearance of her nose because after several decades she has grown accustomed to her face. She wants a nose to fit her face. She does not wish her friends to know she has had a rhinoplasty, at least this is what she says before surgery. On her hidden agenda might be a desire for a more dramatic effect and she might surprise you by saying that you did too little because nobody noticed. The older patient should understand that her tissues are less firm and tip definition is thus harder to achieve. More than in someone younger, subsequent drooping of the tip is likely unless you take precautions against this at surgery. Often a middle-aged woman will consult you for her aging face and eyelids and, in passing, ask about a rhinoplasty—with the comment that she has "always hated" her nose. In my experience, she may settle on an eyelidplasty or facelift but not the rhinoplasty. It is as if she has become re-signed to the nose but not to the recent effects of aging. Some patients have said that a rhinoplasty "at my age is a little ridiculous," but they have little difficulty in accepting facial surgery since many of their friends have had it. That is as common at their age as rhinoplasty was when they were in their teens.

Since these patients are older, a careful medical evaluation by an internist is necessary, especially to rule out hypertension or any other cardiovascular abnormality. These patients may be more sensitive to the action of epinephrine in the local anesthetic. In older patients, as Kaye has noted [84], a partial rhinoplasty may accomplish a great deal: that is, rasping the dorsum or refining the tip.

THE MALE PATIENT FOR RHINOPLASTY

I have previously discussed the fact that the male patient who seeks a rhinoplasty for cosmetic reasons is less likely to be satisfied than his female counterpart [78]. A common sequence is operation → dissatisfaction → re-operation → another plastic surgeon for another operation.

I well remember one man who sought more surgery after he had already had five operations by three other doctors. The nose that he desired was that of a youthful French actress (he had brought her picture). I told him frankly that he should avoid further surgery but should see a psychiatrist. I doubt that this ended his quest.

The unhappy man after rhinoplasty is prone to being litigious. Therefore, at the beginning, choose very carefully the male patient for esthetic nasal surgery.

WHAT ABOUT THE CHIN?

In conjunction with rhinoplasty, a frequent procedure is chin augmentation, generally by means of a synthetic implant or by osteotomy and advancement of the lower portion of the anterior mandible. If the patient has asked about fixing a receding chin, then, of course, the issue is clear; discuss it with him or her. Occasionally patients are unaware, at least consciously, of the chin and the dilemma is whether to raise the issue. It is important not to talk patients into an operation for a problem about which they are unconcerned. If something goes wrong, they would be rightfully angry not only because of the complication but the coercion. It is always possible to do the nose first and the chin later, should the patient desire it. Not every patient is prepared for changing both nose and chin at the same time. The surgeon should be careful not to overwhelm this type of individual with further feelings of inadequacy. I have heard a few surgeons say that because it would be offensive to their esthetic sense and their reputation for a patient with a retruding chin just to have the nose done, they would refuse to do the rhinoplasty. This attitude of the surgeon is imperious and inappropriately possessive about what is truly someone else's body. Some surgeons prefer to take photographs and discuss only the nose at the first consultation and then to have the patient return. On that occasion, with pictures, they can tactfully talk about the nose in relation to the rest of the face, especially the chin. The patient can then think about a mentoplasty and can call the surgeon a few weeks later after making a decision.

THE FINANCES

I have previously alluded to a situation that should not be a problem but frequently is. This concerns whether the patient has a true respiratory obstruction from an internal nasal deformity. If, indeed, none exists then it should not be invoked to gain insurance coverage. This basic concept seems to have eluded many practitioners who become more crooked than the septum they call deviated. I have had many patients say, "Dr. ———— told me that he would state that I had a deviated septum and trouble breathing so our insurance would cover the operation and your charges. After all, I have paid the premium for years and never had to use the insurance." My reply is that the patient has been fortunate to have had good health and, further, I would never falsify any document. I usually add that I would not do it for myself and why should I for someone else? I then suggest that they return to that doctor. Usually they do not. They probably feel uneasy with a doctor who would be willing to lie. If they had been completely satisfied with that surgeon, then they would not have made the appointment to see me.

Dr. Michael Gurdin once remarked [74], "No patient ever thanked me for saving him money." He meant that the patients want the best result and to compromise standards to save a few dollars is usually a foolish exchange for both the surgeon and the patient.

Explicitly tell the patient and family whether you charge for a revision and the approximate cost. If you do not expect a fee, let patients know that they will have to pay for the operating room if you do your surgery at the hospital.

MOTHER AND DAUGHTER COMBINATION

Occasionally, a mother and daughter decide that they wish to be "done together." The surgeon may be flattered by the request and may actually enjoy the special situation, which will be discussed throughout the hospital and give him or her momentary and monetary pleasure. However, the negative aspect is that the father, if there is one, may feel that he is a victim of an unholy alliance: daughter, wife, and surgeon. A more practical consideration is who will be home to care for both the daughter and the mother? Will the father, now disenchanted by their plans, be there to help his errant family? With the mother also recovering from surgery will there be that necessary support, emotional and physical, for the daughter in particular?

Another problem is the decision on whom to operate first. Whoever it is, it is advisable not to let the other see that patient immediately after operation because of possible swelling, ecchymosis, bleeding, pain, nausea, or vomiting. An additional consideration is that the daughter will generally recover faster than the mother, who might feel depressed by this difference. Unpleasant feelings of competition might be aroused [47]. In short, I would approach this doubleheader with great caution.

THE SECOND CONSULTATION

As mentioned, I try not to see a prospective patient for rhinoplasty more than once before surgery. The reason is, I admit, a crowded schedule. However, some surgeons routinely do this. In an excellent chapter, for example, Musgrave and Garrett [100] described their practice of taking Kodachromes and, at another appointment, projecting them for the patient and the family with more explanations about the proposed surgery, with emphasis on its limitations. As a method of preoperative communication, it has proved effective and has diminished ambiguity and false hopes. Its disadvantages are the extra time for you and the patient as well as the expense for the patient to make a return trip or to lose a day or part of one at work. The use of a Polaroid camera at the time of the initial consultation does give you photographs that you can then incorporate into your initial and subsequent discussions with the patient and the family. Other techniques to improve communication are to give printed material to the patient before the consultation or afterwards (or both), or to show prepared audiovisual films, or even to furnish photographs on which patients can then draw to give you (and themselves) a better idea of what they want changed. A problem with this tactic is the tacit implication that you will be able surgically to produce what that patient wants. Performing a rhinoplasty is not custom tailoring.

Despite painstaking preparations and discussion, all of us can remember patients whom we should have weeded out, principally because of their quest for perfection or for the unattainable. If the second consultation is to help you decide about the patient's emotional suitability for surgery, you do have the opportunity for more personality probing. Yet this occasion may foster a bond, albeit tenuous, which should never have arisen. It might be then harder for you to say no. You might have done better in following your intuition at the first visit.

Elsewhere, I have discussed the fact that despite the most careful preoperative discussions, along with written and visual material, patients retain surprisingly little and often only that which causes them the least emotional trauma. They screen out the unpleasant. Doctors may do this also.

Correction of Prominent Ears
PATIENTS

Reduction otoplasty is unique in the list of esthetic operations because it attracts generally those of two disparate types: young boys and older women. It is, therefore, an operation whose need crosses barriers of sex and age. In addition to the concern of human beings about their appearance and their desire not to be singled out because of what society considers a displeasing feature, a factor leading patients to seek the surgery is hairstyle. Until recently, little boys, unlike girls of the same age, did not wear their hair long enough to cover their prominent ears. The older woman, who, when younger, may have obscured her unsightly ears with lengthy tresses, may now want to wear her hair short.

Children in your office for reduction otoplasty may be there at their request or that of their parents. Occasionally, parents may bring a child to you when he is only 2 years of age. Surgeons differ concerning the timing of surgery. I prefer to wait until the child wants the operation, usually between the ages of 4 and 6 years, when playmates are quick to fasten on a deviant physical characteristic. The child, whose name the parents have carefully chosen, now becomes "Bat Ears" or "Elephant Head" or something equally inelegant.

If the parents bring the child to you before he realizes that his ears are disagreeably visible, he will feel that the hospitalization and surgery have been imposed unfairly upon him. His willingness to cooperate will be less than if he had asked for the operation himself, and his psychological trauma may be more intense. The parent understandably desires to spare the child peer abuse; perhaps the mother or father had a similar problem for which he or she may have had surgery.

One of the parents may still have prominent ears and may say that "I want the operation to be done now in order to spare him what I had to go through." Occasionally a parent will have a reduction otoplasty soon after the child has had his.

Be certain to know the child as an individual, not only his medical history, with possible allergies, but his interests—that is, preference for TV programs, sports, and so on. It is too easy to forget that this small patient is a person and not just a member of an amorphous species called children.

The older patient, usually a woman, may now want to "set the ears back" because, as mentioned, she may wish a different hairstyle. Usually, the patient will say something like, "I have hated my ears since I was a kid. I'm tired of wearing my hair like this and now that my children are older, I thought I would do something for myself." Compared to facelift, eyelidplasty, rhinoplasty, breast augmentation, and breast reduction, this procedure does not evoke much response in the spouse. He may be concerned about the cost but not about her safety or his reactions to the physical transformation. The ears are a sexually neutral area of the body. Of course, with more sex manuals appearing each day, one cannot predict the next focus.

PHYSICAL EXAMINATION
Since not all ears are alike, even those in the same individual, your examination must determine the specific aspect for correction. Note the presence or absence of cupping and asymmetry. Test also for gross hearing so that you could not be accused of causing an auditory impairment. This is not the place to list the numerous abnormalities that can occur among the many hillocks and valleys of the external ear. You should know, however, what operation you will do before you get to the operating room; for example, reduce the concha and/or retroflex the antihelix, or something else.

INFORMING THE PATIENT
For the young child, reduction otoplasty usually requires general anesthesia on an outpatient basis or during a day or two in the hospital. In the older child or adult, the operation is usually done under local anesthesia on an outpatient basis.

The patient and family should not expect absolute symmetry

but should expect no more abnormal projection to the ears. If, in your experience, two or three percent of patients have recurrence of their condition, so inform the patient and the family. Infection is uncommon, as is hematoma, but each is possible.

Scars are generally imperceptible but keloids do occur. The sharp edge of the antihelix upsets the surgeon but rarely the patient or family. What truly causes disappointment and anger is not getting the ears back far enough.

The patient and the family must know what type of pain to expect. It is not a procedure free of discomfort; because it is far from life-threatening, this operation may be passed off to the patient as minimal and the patient will be surprised by the amount of pain he or she might experience.

Also tell patients how long they are expected to wear a head dressing and whether you will also require them to have an ear-head band at night (and for how long). The bulky, warm dressing around the head can be very uncomfortable during the summer, when many children (not at school) and adults (vacation time and their children away at camp) have it done.

In some states, not the majority, insurance will defray the bills of the surgeon and the hospital. The patient and the family must clearly understand their financial obligations, particularly if there is no third-party coverage.

The impression of many surgeons is that the popularity of this procedure is declining, perhaps due more to the current hairstyles than to the incidence of the condition, the economic realities of our society, or social indifference.

In dealing with children, explain the procedure clearly: Do not overwhelm them with details but do not minimize or omit unpleasantries (see pp. 161–165). The child, like any patient, will want to know about pain. You may reassure the child that he or she will not experience pain during the operation but afterwards, and that medicine can make it better. If there is a pediatric ward in the hospital or, indeed, the child will be going to a children's hospital, you can describe the environment and even arrange for him to visit before admission. Always offer to answer questions after you have finished talking and tell the child that should he or she have any further questions or any worries, you would be happy to hear

91

from him. If you have to communicate with the parents, a little note to the child also will make him or her feel better, letting him know that you think of him as an individual and not simply an extension of his parents. Hopefully, your habit is to see all patients the afternoon or evening before surgery; telling the child that you will see him soon after his admission to the hospital will decrease his anxiety.

Eyelidplasty and Facelift

Time was beginning to walk across the face.
ROGER KAHN
The Boys of Summer

They aren't making mirrors the way they used to.
TALLULAH BANKHEAD

PATIENTS
Patients for these procedures are most likely to be white, middle- or upper-class women (1 in 10 is a man) between the ages of 45 and 55. Characteristically, they are energetic and active socially and professionally. The patient is not usually one of the "idle rich." Having been considered attractive throughout her life, she fears losing what has been an important asset [57]. One woman quoted her mother as saying, "A beautiful woman dies twice." Most who come for an eyelidplasty and facelift do not want to dissimulate their age but to reaffirm to themselves and perhaps to others that they are still youthful, optimistic, and effective [64]. Many say that they do not desire to look much younger but want to avoid appearing much older. They still think of themselves as more youthful than they are chronologically. For some, a sagging face is symbolic of life's inexorable downhill course. They do not want to see their life contracting coffinlike around them; they are in your office to rid themselves of the daily reminders of decay.

Surgery for the aging face is frequently sought after a recent loss, such as separation, divorce, death, removal of body part (mastectomy, hysterectomy; see p. 45), or termination of psychotherapy. The woman in her mid-40s may be either in the menopause or facing it. Losses start overcoming gains: Her body has aged; her children have left; her husband's attentions may have waned; at work, she may feel excluded by those younger; there is now less sand in the hourglass. For some, the facelift is an active means of coping with life; they can have a facelift even though they cannot keep their children from leaving home. The facelift may be a passport to a new pattern of living or to the resumption of an old career, perhaps interrupted by marriage and child rearing.

In our society and in much of the world, the woman suffers from what Sontag has called "the double standard of aging." Women are penalized more for aging than are men. "Aging means a humiliating process of gradual sexual disqualification . . . . Aging is much more a social judgment than a biological eventuality [137]."

The process of aging is generally imperceptible on a day-by-day basis; it proceeds somewhat slowly but not necessarily at the same pace. There are, however, what the French term *crises d'âge*—when suddenly a person seems to age rapidly. Many patients say, "Just recently, I look so old. I don't mind getting older, but not this fast." That observation may coincide with an emotional trauma. Many have correctly recognized that their tendency to aging is familial and resent this inherited trait, especially if an older sister has escaped it or her mother has had it. Commonly I hear a patient say: "I dread getting to look like my mother." She resents the unpleasant irony of beginning to resemble the person toward whom she has such deep ambivalence.

Many women wish to appear young for professional reasons, as in the performing arts, or because of a liaison with someone younger. Statistically these patients are in the minority. Most seeking an eyelidplasty and facelift want to lessen the visible evidence of time's passage in order to improve their self-image.

The patient may feel ashamed about having cosmetic surgery. Often, she has had to wage her battle alone. Friends may consider her foolish; her husband may call her "crazy"; and her family doctor may be strongly opposed. The following letter is typical of that kind of physician: punitive, rigid, and unsympathetic.

Dear Doctor Goldwyn:
    When I saw Lisa Albert a few weeks ago, I was surprised to hear her express an interest in a facelift.

She is a lovely, little old lady, rather childish in her behavior and lost since her husband's death several years ago, drifts from one relative to another and is an extremely passive and dependent lady.

As far as her medical history, there is no contraindication to the surgical procedure; however, it would seem to be a radical step to satisfy this masochistic need.

She did have a rhytidectomy and was very pleased with the result. A close relative, previously skeptical, reported that it "did her a world of good. I was surprised."

One patient termed the entire process of obtaining a facelift a "lonely vigil." In a world where the haves are reminded of the have-nots, she may feel even more guilty because she is spending money (often her husband's), since cosmetic surgery and the associated hospitalization generally are not covered by insurance. Many apologize for taking the doctor's "valuable time" and for occupying a hospital bed "meant for sick people." The patient considers the operation for improving the aging face to be an enhancement. She will accommodate to the "new look" since it is really the old look—the way she was.

Other patients, however, come for a facelift/eyelidplasty as a way of beginning life anew, the operation being emotionally a reparation for damages suffered. I remember a 42-year-old woman whose daughter had died following a four-year battle with leukemia. "Now I can do something for myself," she declared.

INITIAL CONSULTATION

At the first visit, it is essential for the surgeon to know what the patient wishes and what type of individual he or she is. Unlike the man wishing a rhinoplasty, men desiring eyelidplasty and facelift are usually stable and as satisfied with their result as their female counterparts. In my experience, the man actually seems easier to please in these cases, and is not more psychologically ill as others have reported [78].

Someone observed, and many would agree, that cosmetic surgery would be easy if it were not for the patients. By that, we are acknowledging the fact that technically, though this type of surgery is exacting, it does not require extraordinary talents. The problem is that patients are often demanding and fussy about results. It is probably unreasonable for us to expect that someone who was sufficiently concerned about his or her looks to undertake surgery will, after operation, not care about a little wrinkle or bulge. What I try to do during the first visit is to avoid operating upon the patient who cannot stand imperfection because, frankly, most patients after facelift and eyelidplasty will have imperfections; the flawless result is seen more often in slides at meetings and in articles in journals than in one's own office—at least, in mine. I have reviewed the charts of my patients who have had lingering dissatisfaction with the outcome of these procedures. Statistically, they represent 8 percent of all patients but emotionally in terms of their impact on the surgeon, they seem to be a much larger number. In every instance, my secretaries and/or I had a presentiment that this patient might be "difficult." Most were hard to please in other spheres of life; at least that had been my impression. What most surgeons do not know is how many emotionally difficult patients have fared well in our care. We remember the problem patients but forget those from whom expected trouble did not arise. There are some patients for whom a home run—not a triple—is essential to success and, more than that, the ball must be hit exactly in right center field. As I get older, I prefer not to accept such challenges. Unlike in fishing, the one that gets away in plastic surgery may be a blessing for you.

Baker has said, "The object of the operation should be to improve appearance not to make the patient happy if she is sad to begin with. You both will likely end up sad [6]."

In your history taking, be certain to inquire about general health, including present or past psychotherapy, previous operations and emotional reactions to them, allergies, and medications, especially aspirin-containing compounds.

PHYSICAL EXAMINATION
I always ask the patient to indicate while holding a mirror what she or he would like improved. In general, in comparison with men, women are more conscious of the skin redundancy and sagging of their upper lids than of their lower lids. That is likely due to their using eye makeup, with a liner in the upper fold.

Frequently, the patient wants only her neck done and even though she might benefit also from an eyelidplasty, it is advisable not to extend the scope of the surgery. The patient's face, like every other body part, is hers; she may allow us to operate but we are not given a carte blanche to pursue our trade wherever we wish. A patient and a surgeon do better to undertake less than to try for more. Additional surgery is always possible later but you cannot take back what you have already done. Nowhere else in medicine are Aristotle's words more true than in cosmetic surgery [4]. "It is no part of a physician's . . . business to use either persuasion or compulsion upon the patient." The procedure you might add to the patient's list is likely to be the one that will have a complication.

Occasionally, a true dilemma exists. A patient, for example, who wants only the upper lids done may thereby accentuate the aging of the lower lids (painting-just-one-room-in-a-house syndrome), making her face as a whole look worse by comparison. However, if carried to absurdity, an upper eyelidplasty would lead to a lower eyelidplasty, a face and neck lift, a mastopexy, an abdominoplasty, a thigh lift, and, perhaps, a rhinoplasty. The patient's desires and your common sense should establish the direction and limits of the surgery.

An important point in the preoperative examination of a patient for an eyelidplasty or a facelift is to note facial asymmetry, in repose and in smiling. Is there any weakness of any branch of the facial nerve (possible evidence of Bell's palsy)? Whatever differences exist between one side of the face and the other, and there usually are some, should be shown to the patient by means of a mirror and/or photographs. Postoperatively, that person might expect more symmetry than he or she ever had or could ever have. It is interesting to observe how little error patients can tolerate after operation and how much imperfection they had managed to live with before.

Although this book is not intended to be a text on plastic surgery, I think it is important to emphasize the need for a thorough eye examination, if not by you, then by an ophthalmologist. Be certain also that the patient, especially if older, has had a thorough examination by an ophthalmologist within the past six months or year. I always write the eye specialist about the contemplated surgery in order to obtain reports about his or her findings and suggestions. You should test at least gross vision: ability to read with and without glasses. Also evaluate the patient's ability to lacrimate in order to detect the actual or potential "dry eye."

WRINKLES OR SAGGING OR BOTH?

For someone whose face has the Gucci bag look, dermabrasion or chemical peel in addition to or instead of a surgical rhytidectomy may be what the patient needs, particularly if she minds the wrinkles more than the sagging. She might benefit optimally from both procedures, staged to avoid the application of phenol to skin just undermined. Occasionally, a patient will refuse a chemical peel because she fears scarring, a remote possibility, or dislikes a permanent change in pigment, a likely event. For want of something better, you and the patient may settle for just the surgical lift. Despite your candid and thorough explanation of the limitations of the rhytidectomy alone and her declaration that she understands what you are saying but she will be grateful for "whatever you can do for me," you both are sinking into the slippery and steep-walled pit that you have dug for yourselves.

E. N., a 63-year-old sales manager, widow, and former solarphile, had marked wrinkling of her cheeks and forehead, and around her mouth. She also had moderate jowls and prominent platysmal bands in her neck. Her principal concern was her cheek creases, which, I explained, would be managed best by a chemical peel. Since I do not do this, I offered to refer her. When she understood that the procedure could be followed by scarring (a rare event) and permanent change in pigment (a common occurrence), she decided to have a surgical lift for the improvement she could expect with regard to her jowls and neck.

SHE: Even though a peel and lift would be the best, a lift by itself would help me, wouldn't it?

I: Yes, but only mildly.

SHE: What would you do?

I: That's for you to decide. But why don't you at least get an opinion from someone who frequently does the chemical peel?

SHE: You say that no one can guarantee that there will not be scarring?

I: Yes, but scarring is not common after a peel.

SHE: But you also said that my skin may not keep the same color it has now if I have the chemical applied.

I: True, but you will look better with many of the lines and wrinkles gone.

SHE: Well, if you don't do the chemical peel, there must be others who also don't do it and there must be reasons for this. So, I have made up my mind. I want a facelift and I will have to be satisfied with any improvement it will give me even though it may not be as good as if I also had the chemical treatment.

A few weeks after an uneventful facelift and when the swelling regressed and the lines reappeared, she seemed subdued, evidently depressed, and said, "Even though you told me that I wouldn't get a fantastic improvement, I honestly thought it would be more than this. My friends can't believe I ever had anything done."

I again offered her the opportunity to supplement the facelift by a chemical peel but she refused for the same reasons as before. Only now, she considers the small gain from the surgery as a loss because of her large outlay—physically, emotionally, and financially.

The lesson from this patient is clear and it has relevance to all elective surgical situations, not just the instance of the patient with the wrinkled face: It is better to do nothing than something of dubious value. At best, it will never succeed relative to the patient's desires and expectations. Painting the living room when the dining room really needs it rarely satisfies a customer.

INFORMING THE PATIENT

In a chronological sequence, I take the patient through the contemplated surgery. For those wishing an eyelidplasty, I discuss the mechanisms of outpatient surgery (at the hospital); the use of local anesthesia with intravenous supplementation; the expected pain; the length of the procedure (an hour and a half); the need for someone to drive them home; the regimen of bed rest, head elevation, and iced dressings to the eyes for 24 hours; the return visit to the office for suture removal in three to five days; and the expected resumption of normal activities—in the home or at the office—in three to seven days after operation depending upon the nature and setting of the job.

With the patient holding a mirror, I indicate the incisions and inform him or her about the inevitability of scars, but say that hopefully they will not be noticeable at conversation distance. I do emphasize, however, that wound healing is unpredictable and that scarring might be prominent, red, and thick. I also tell patients about the small probability of infection and hematoma. I inform them also about the much smaller chance of blindness in one or both eyes. The patient and the family must understand that although an eyelidplasty is not a major operation, like a gastrectomy, it is a surgical event subject to unpredictable occurrences—one of which is blindness. Admittedly, this event is uncommon but I never do a bilateral lower eyelidplasty in a patient with vision in only one eye.

With every patient I clearly stress the limitations of the surgery: not to expect every wrinkle to disappear but to anticipate significant lessening of skin redundancy and prominent bags. I tell each patient that swelling and ecchymosis will last two to three weeks but that he or she must wait six to nine months for a near-final result. To the question of how long the surgical improvement will last, I say that the lift may stall the aging process but it never halts it. In general, the worse the problem, the longer the benefit. Even the best-executed operation can produce only a minimal effect if the problem is minimal. The patient is told that aging and the surgical results vary from individual to individual, depending upon genetic factors, past and present, and future health and other variables beyond human control. Some patients have the misconception that suddenly one morning they will wake and have their face "drop." This fantasy may reflect their guilt about trying to thwart nature. Since I hospitalize patients having facelifts, I explain the admitting process. Fortunately, nurses and personnel are not now so punitive toward these patients as they once were. In some hospitals, patients for cosmetic surgery have been treated as intruders.

For those having a facelift alone or with an eyelidplasty, I demonstrate the planned incisions around the ears, into the hairline, and possibly under the chin if something has to be done for the neck through this approach. I mention many of the things that I have already discussed for an eyelidplasty. In addition, I tell the patient about the possibility of damage to the facial nerve, a surgical event more often discussed than observed but one that can occur, especially as the procedure now involves more being done to the fat of the cheeks and neck and to the platysma. These patients must understand that they may feel an unpleasant constriction and numbness in their neck for a few months but usually these sensations disappear.

Some patients may have excessively redundant skin of their lids, cheeks, and neck; I tell them that a secondary procedure may be necessary in six to twelve months to improve the initial results. Patients having a facelift want to know the length of the operation (three to four hours), the type of anesthesia (local and intravenous), the duration of hospitalization (two days), whether their hair is shaved (no, except only to make an incision), when they can go to the hairdresser (six days for a shampoo; twelve days for color), whether they will go home with a bandage (no), when the stitches are removed (three to five days for the lids; seven to ten days for sutures in front of the ears and ten days for those behind), how long the swelling and ecchymosis will last (two to three weeks, but the final result will take six to nine months to be appreciated), when they can use makeup (to the face, around five days, but not over the incisions; false eyelashes, six days after operation). Various surgeons will answer these questions differently but the important point is to answer them or to raise them if the patient has not thought of them.

I also tell patients that it is not unusual to have a mild depression for a few days after operation. This is due not only to the patient's seeing herself in a contused, unnatural condition but also to the metabolic response to surgery—initial euphoria followed by a downward mood swing. Moreover, the fact that these operations are done under local anesthesia with intravenous medication does not make them "minor" procedures, as far as the patient's response is concerned. The challenge to soma and psyche is greater than the patient expects and the surgeon appreciates. Numbness and paresthesias will add to discomfort and depression.

Fees, of course, must also be discussed—the cost of your services as well as that of the hospital, operating room, anesthesia (or of the office if the surgery is being performed there). Make clear that third-party coverage is usually unavailable for cosmetic surgery and for any complications such as hematoma and infection.

IN THE HOSPITAL

Frequently a patient for cosmetic surgery will ask as you leave her room, "You are going to make me gorgeous and beautiful, aren't you?" This plea from a 55-year-old woman comes after all your disclaimers. Especially at the end of the day, it is tempting to say "Of course," and with a wave of the hand, walk out of the room. Do not literally take the easy way out. Return to the bedside and sit down. What you should say in response is something like, "It would be easier for me to leave the room and simply tell you 'yes, I will.' However, the reality is that while I expect you will be improved, there will be no magical transformation. After all, like the tailor, I can work only with the cloth that I have. I do understand your desire to look much better and I certainly will try my best." Again, this tack allows you to reinforce the reality principle. If, indeed, this dialogue with the patient leads you to feel that she still is expecting a Ponce de Leon transformation, perhaps it is better to part company then, even though she has been admitted for surgery.

DURING OPERATION.   Remarks about technique belong in other books. The only point I wish to make here is that since the patient is not usually completely asleep, you and your assistants, as well as the nurses, must be very careful about what you say to each other. Since the operation lasts three to four hours, there is ample time to let down your guard to the emotional discomfort of the patient. For example, one patient recalled that I had said to my assistant, "The bleeding is more than I expected." The patient said that she wanted to question me at that point but had expressive aphasia, frequently seen with neuroleptic anesthesia accompanying local infiltration. To the observer, the patient seemed completely relaxed and happy; her inner turmoil was not apparent.

AFTER OPERATION

Although most patients having eyelidplasty and facelift will be satisfied if they have been properly selected, this does not guarantee that all patients will be beaming with gratitude. Those who have had the operation not just to look younger but to recapture youth will be disappointed. Their lease on life has not been extended. The plastic surgeon who carefully questions patients following the procedure will detect more depression than had been suspected or has been commonly reported. As mentioned, this emotional letdown usually passes but it may persist. Despite what you have said, the patient may have forgotten that she would get depressed and despite your telling her not to expect too much from the procedure, she may have anticipated a miraculous transformation, an immediate turning back of the clock by 20 years—without swelling or ecchymosis.

During her recovery, the patient has probably had to hide from all but her closest friends. Only her hairdresser knows. As one patient said, "I learned to sit in the first row in church so I could get out first and also to sit with my thumb under my chin (hiding the incision)."

For many women seeking a facelift or eyelidplasty, the surgeon is the hired hand. He has been asked to do a job just as she might have requested a mechanic to repair her auto. When the result is good, the patient is pleased but not grateful, unlike the patient who has had a musculocutaneous flap for a debilitating chronic ulcer of the lower leg or the patient who has undergone a much-needed reduction mammoplasty. Aside from their general disenchantment, patients may be greatly upset if a complication or unfavorable result ensues. Do not expect them to accept this turn of events with equanimity. Although you have told them about its possibility, most patients will not consider it seriously. If they did, they probably never would have pursued their request for the operation. Therefore, when a complication does occur, they feel wronged and may be extremely angry at what they consider your "incompetence." How to manage this trying situation is discussed later (see pp. 168–176). A further difficulty is that since insurance does not usually defray the cost of complications, they feel even more unhappy and resentful. If we were in their position, we would probably react the same way.

If indeed the patient seems to have a severe postoperative psychological disturbance, do not wait long to call a psychiatrist.

Often, it is a reactive depression that will pass, hopefully, with appropriate therapy or even with time alone. The problem is often how to get the patient who needs the psychiatrist to the psychiatrist.

In conclusion, the eyelidplasty and facelift can be satisfying operations for patients as well as surgeons. However, remember that a principal objective of the initial consultation is to identify that patient who is not a good candidate for this surgery, either because of what she wants, what she has, or how she is [119]. Again, my advice is to select that patient *who can tolerate imperfection* and truly understands the limitations of the operation.

THE OPINIONS OF OTHERS AS A DETERMINANT OF POSTOPERATIVE SATISFACTION.   After eyelidplasty and facelift, more than anywhere else in esthetic plastic surgery, the opinions of others, even strangers, may greatly influence the patient's satisfaction or dissatisfaction with the anatomical outcome [120]. This is true to some degree after rhinoplasty with regard to the judgment of the parent, particularly the mother and peers. My observations suggest that the friends of the adolescent girl are usually more supportive than those of the middle-aged woman, who is extremely vulnerable to the opinions of her friends, especially those of the same sex. Their approbation or disapproval is usually more important to her than that of her husband. Because she may have undertaken her surgery with his opposition or grudging consent, his opinion is not now important since it never was.

Even though the patient sought the operation by herself and presumably for herself, she is very much aware of the reaction of those around her. Just at the time she desperately wants their support, her friends may impale her by their verbal thrusts.

"You certainly are swollen. Will it ever go away under your chin?"
"You really look funny."
"Your eyes don't match."
"How come Betty looks so much better than you and you went to the same surgeon?" (Betty may be six months postoperative and your patient, only three weeks.)

"I told you that you should have gone to somebody else."
"After seeing what you look like, I'd never have it done."

How apt the line from the Old Testament, "I was wounded in the house of my friends" (Zech. 13:6).

The patient's "friend" may resent her likely change for the better. Perhaps that friend may have wanted the operation but lacked the money or courage or both. She may also fear that her husband will now find her rejuvenated friend more attractive than she. It is probably true that a good friend helps you in distress but a better friend helps you in success.

The surgeon cannot insulate a patient from the barbs of those close to her. However, he or she can support her recovery from injury and can point out the possible psychodynamics responsible for a "friend's" behavior. It takes considerable control for you, as a surgeon, not to become angry at the patient's friends for making such remarks and for withholding much-needed succor.

When the patient is at a low ebb, she may not be able to deal with distressing situations that she has previously managed fairly well—for example, an unhappy relationship with her husband or a child. In addition, the operation itself may become a focus of generalized hostility. The patient in response to the pressures may complain of insomnia, pain in the face and neck, and unhappiness with the result of her procedure. By listening to the patient and by not running away from her (with the excuse that many others are waiting), you may be able to sort the causative from the incidental factors. You may then be able to give the patient a perspective on her problems. Your reassurance will help restore her confidence and temporarily wounded self-esteem.

As Goin has written [54], many people who have esthetic surgery are those

with high personal standards of performance, the need to deny their wishes to be cared for, and an obsession with their independence. They feel guilty and down when they are not meeting these standards. Patients find they are not able to function at their preoperative capacity for a few days. If they were ill with cancer, this might seem acceptable, but following elective operation it is intolerable. The guilt about self-indulgence is already at a high level and consequently it is important to carry on at home as if nothing has happened. The mother of six feels it is important to be up and ready to go at 6:30 A.M., getting her children off to school efficiently, clean, cook, or, if she works, go off to work as usual. When she finds herself unable to tackle these tasks with her normal vigor, she is struck with a sense of inadequacy and guilt over inability and sense of depression.

Patients with that type of personality are most prone to depression, which sometimes the surgeon can relieve, but which occasionally does require a psychotherapist.

Breast Augmentation
PATIENTS

From a psychiatric evaluation of patients undergoing augmentation mammoplasty, Gifford [51] concluded that many had

unhappy childhoods, experience of loss or maternal deprivation, and conflicts in identification with parents. They tended to make early marriages, in which they played a submissive or frankly masochistic role . . . many described longstanding feelings of inferiority or low self-esteem, and several described periods of clinical depression. The "typical" breast augmentation patient seemed to have reached an emotional turning point in her life, when she had decided against having more children and was seeking a new direction, increased self-assertiveness, some kind of personality change. In these women, the breasts had come to represent something more than sexual attractiveness, because their breasts were their representation of an ideal self, real or imagined. This was an image of themselves as they were at some former time or as they had hoped to be, an ideal self which they had been deprived of or lost through hardship, childbearing or the vicissitudes of life. The operation represented the restitution of this loss, the restoration of an ideal or former self.

Other studies have documented depression, low self-esteem in general and as a woman in particular, as well as hysterical traits in patients requesting breast enlargement [134]. However, Shipley, O'Donnel, and Bader [131], who used control groups of small and average-busted women, concluded that their patients for augmentation were psychologically healthy although they placed greater emphasis on physical attractiveness and "modern or revealing" dress. Their data did not support the findings of others [9, 38] that women for this procedure suffered from low self-esteem or poor general body image. Also, there was no evidence of depression, social malfunction, or a higher incidence of either major gynecological surgery or psychiatric counseling.

To state the incontestably obvious, these patients feel inadequate about their breasts, specifically, their size. When surgery gives them larger breasts, they are almost always satisfied with the result [77, 107, 134]. Thus plastic surgeons can continue performing an operation that in 30 to 50 percent of patients produces an undesirable result because of unnatural firmness and contour. In 17 years of practice, I have been asked by only one patient to remove the implants. In this individual, the reason was not capsular contracture but religion, the fear that God would punish her by causing breast cancer for having altered her body. In her case, I had had enough misgivings before surgery to ask for an evaluation by a psychiatrist whose advice was to proceed.

When one asks a patient why she wants this operation now, the usual response is that the small size of her breasts has always "bothered" her and "finally I want to do something about it." Some will complain that buying clothes is a "hassle." Passing through the mind of this male surgeon is the thought that taking the risk of surgery with its attendant pain to change one's body shape just to buy clothes seems astounding. However, the real reason for having the surgery is much deeper and more important than the issue of shopping for clothes.

Another group of patients will say openly that their adolescent daughter is "built better" than they are—which is patently upsetting to them.

Patients who are married are frequently accompanied by their husbands, who seem perplexed by their wives' behavior, since the size of their breasts has never been a barrier to their physical attraction. However, the discussion of this problem has usually been long-standing and over the years the husband has finally consented but unenthusiastically. He is concerned justifiably with the danger of the operation, its cost, and its possible carcinogenic effects. He is also hopeful but somewhat dubious that the augmentation will satisfy the patient's expectations and make her feel "good about herself." Only rarely does the patient seek the operation because of a request by a man. In that situation, it is unwise to be the surgeon who implements her acquiescence and masochism.

Frequently, women for augmentation mammoplasty are in

transition—between marriages, affairs, or careers. They are undertaking surgery to start life anew by correcting something that disturbed them emotionally for many years and that now might make them less able to establish a gratifying and easy relationship with a new man [99].

As a group, these patients are less perfectionistic than those for eyelidplasty, facelift, or rhinoplasty. There is, however, a small subgroup who constitute a cause for concern; those who upon physical examination have normal size breasts, but who nevertheless insist that they are "too small." Under these circumstances, I suggest that they not have surgery but, if they insist, I refer them to another plastic surgeon.

Inquiries concerning previous pregnancies and nursing and possible future pregnancies with nursing, as well as family history of breast cancer should be routine. Is the patient prone to recurrent pain or "lumps" in the breast? Has she ever had biopsies? Does she regularly examine her breasts?

PHYSICAL EXAMINATION

That 1 in 15 women in the United States will develop breast cancer at some point in her life should be sufficiently sobering to the surgeon to perform a thorough breast examination. In addition, for every patient 35 or older, I order mammograms unless recent ones (within the past nine months) are available. In your exam, look for breast asymmetry and if present, point it out to the patient. Its presence may change your usual operative plan and choice of implant. The patient's body build is important. Examine and photograph the patient not only from the front but from the back in an upright and flexed position to detect and document scoliosis and chest deformities, such as pectus excavatum.

INFORMING THE PATIENT

Size. Most patients have a definite idea of what they want for size. Sometimes their expectations are unrealistic. For example, I recall one petite woman who wished to go from a 34-A to a 34-D. Not only did she lack sufficient soft tissue to harbor such implants but the esthetic result would have been poor—even bizarre. Despite my explanation, including a statement that such massive prostheses would predispose her to abnormal firmness and contour, she persisted. I suggested that she consult another plastic surgeon who might comply with her wishes.

In general, I use prostheses (suprapectoral) no greater than 150 to 165 cc, since most of my patients wish to fill a B cup. Seemingly, the more intellectual the patient, the more anxiety she has about becoming too large. She is usually concerned that others will note a drastic modification. This sentiment is particularly true of high school teachers who fear their class's response. In 17 years of practice I have had perhaps four or five patients who were disappointed because I had not made them larger. In a couple of patients, I did make a mistake because I had not taken into account their height, broad shoulders, and the laxity of their breast and chest tissue. In those situations, I offer to exchange the implants at no charge but they are responsible for the hospital expenses. All these patients declined further surgery because they did "not feel like going through that operation and pain again." Furnas' suggestion [48] to let the patient make the final decision about size by seeing herself in a mirror during surgery is worthwhile; however, one must remember that she is under the influence of medication.

From articles and presentations at meetings, it is apparent the choice of size varies widely according to the desires of the patient and the doctor. However, there is also a geographical factor. In the western and southwestern parts of the country, my colleagues are routinely inserting implants twice as large as I use. Perhaps the "wide-open spaces" increase expectations.

BREAST HYPOPLASIA AND PECTUS EXCAVATUM.   For these patients, a decision has to be made about correcting the pectus excavatum or leaving it and augmenting only the breasts. Sometimes, a breast augmentation will make more noticeable the pectus deformity. In other patients, however, augmenting the breasts and placing the implants medially will help obscure the pectus. Some patients will require one operation for correction of the pectus and another for the augmentation; in others, everything can be done at the same time. Usually a custom-made moulage for the pectus is mandatory. The important point about these patients is to consider their entire breast and chest as a totality and to realize that their surgical problems are not solved by the usual, relatively simple, breast augmentation.

HEMATOMA AND INFECTION. These complications can follow any operation. In my experience the likelihood of expanding hematoma requiring immediate evacuation is about two percent. For that reason, patients who live more than one and one-half hours' drive from the hospital are advised to stay overnight nearby. A hematoma is an unfortunate happening not only because it imposes on the patient more physical stress, but also because it adds to her financial burden since most insurance plans will not defray the hospital charges for the treatment of any complication following a cosmetic procedure that itself was not initially covered. Needless to mention, your services should be free. The patient may require general anesthesia for adequate management of her anxiety as well as for operating ease to remove the hematoma and to control bleeding—a painful process. Also, a 24-hour hospitalization will probably be necessary. Surgeons who operate in their offices have an advantage since they can offer their facility free of charge but mobilizing nurses and possibly an anesthesiologist at night may be impractical or impossible, and a hospital will be needed. The patient must be told in the initial consultation that she will be responsible for the expenses arising from complications. Discuss specifically the sequence of events should a hematoma occur.

Infection, fortunately, is uncommon—less than one percent incidence in my experience; but the patient must understand that it can occur and that it is not always susceptible to antibiotics [30]. In that event, removal of the implant(s) with a later attempt at augmentation will be required.

INCISIONS, APPROACH, AND SCARS. Whatever your surgical approach, a patient must know it. She must also be told of the possibility that her scars might be red and thick even though usually they are not. You must frankly inform the patient that a man might notice her scars even if they are located in the areola. Inform the patient also where the implant will lie in relation to the breast—under or over the muscle. This information will be important for her to relate to other doctors who examine her.

ABILITY TO NURSE.   I have had many patients nurse following an augmentation mammoplasty performed either through the inframammary or the intraareolar approach. Some patients, however, especially if they have had no children, prefer the inframammary because it will theoretically disrupt the breast tissue less than an operation via the areola. Preferences should be heeded even though data are lacking to support that contention. If a patient is planning to become pregnant soon and wishes to nurse, it would be wiser to defer the operation until the child has been weaned.

TYPE OF IMPLANT.   Most surgeons have chosen from the bewildering assortment of implants one or two types that they prefer for most patients having symmetrical mammary hypoplasia. I show the patient a prototype of the gel implant I use, taking care to state that "this will not be your size," if it is not. Since I also use inflatables, less now than before because of late deflation, I also discuss this alternative with patients. Many have heard that the inflatables give a softer breast and, indeed, several reports have confirmed this impression. However, I emphasize that no prosthesis can give a predictably normal breast in every instance.

FIRMNESS AND ABNORMAL CONTOUR.   These unfavorable results are the principal problems with augmentation mammoplasty. In my experience, about 25 percent of patients have unusual firmness in one or both breasts postoperatively. I have not yet begun to place the implants routinely under the pectoral muscle. The patient must understand that thick capsules and contracture can occur, no matter what and where the implant or who the surgeon. I tell them that steroids and/or antibiotics will be instilled into the dissected pocket but their value is controversial. I also say that occasionally steroids may cause skin atrophy and descent of the prosthesis.

Patients want to know what can be done about abnormal firmness. I explain that manual compression in the office can reduce the problem but only in about half the instances. Surgical release is possible but I inform patients that many women may be left with persistent firmness, even after one or two more capsulotomies. Sometimes, it is then necessary to place the implant under the muscle should severe capsular contracture persist.

I tell the prospective patients that many patients who have had firmness have chosen to live with it, unless they are bothered by inability to lie flat on their abdomen or by discomfort during intercourse or by their general feelings of disappointment with the abnormal shape and feel of their augmented breasts. The patient is told also that since the operation of augmentation seems to give the woman satisfaction because of the size of her breasts, only a very small percentage of patients who have firmness will elect to have more than a manual capsulotomy and some even refuse that.

The patient must understand also that since you cannot guarantee a normal flowing and feeling breast, a man might know that she has "had something done" even if he does not see the scars. For some patients a photograph of a patient with moderately severe bilateral and unilateral capsular contracture is necessary to get your point across if you sense that the patient cannot comprehend this kind of problem.

COLD SENSATION. Many patients, including some of my own, have complained that they were not properly informed about the fact that their breasts would feel cold, particularly during the winter. This has more relevance, of course, for those in New England than in a tropical climate. This is not usually a primary complaint, but when other things go wrong after augmentation, the patient will likely mention it—as another instance of being imperfectly apprised of the consequences of this procedure.

SENSATION. For many years, it was not generally appreciated that augmentation mammoplasty altered sensation of the skin of the breast, the areola, and the nipple [29]. Usually the problem is hypoesthesia and that is mild and transient; yet I have had patients who admit, if questioned carefully, that they still are "numb" in the area of the nipple and areola, and objective testing with a voltimeter* confirms it. Usually, however, their erotic responses may even be heightened because they feel more secure about themselves and more relaxed during sex. These changes in sensation have occurred in equal frequency with the areola and inframammary approach.

PAIN.   Since people vary in their tolerance for pain, you must establish whether a particular patient can be operated on under local anesthesia (with intravenous supplementation) as an outpatient. In my experience, about 95 percent of women can be managed in this way and prefer it; it allows them to resume almost immediately their usual life-style; to preserve relative anonymity by going home and not meeting friends in the hospital; and, of course, it significantly lowers costs. However, some patients may be very needle shy and susceptible to physical pain. They should be given general anesthesia on an outpatient basis, if indicated, and not be made to feel inferior because they cannot tolerate or do not want local anesthesia. To allay their feelings of guilt about more expense and their sense of inferiority, perhaps long-standing because of their small-sized breasts, I point out that each human being has his or her own strengths and weaknesses and that she might tolerate emotional stresses of another sort far better than other patients and some of her friends, for example. Not everyone is or even should be a Spartan. I repeat Socrates' admonition: Know thyself. In general, women who have had natural childbirth or who practice yoga and/or transcendental meditation are good candidates for outpatient surgery and local anesthesia.

POSSIBLE FUTURE BREAST CANCER.   Most patients, certainly their husbands, will ask about possible carcinogenic effects of augmentation mammoplasty. To this question, I reply that so far no study has shown that this procedure increases or decreases the woman's chance for developing a breast malignancy. Usually an intelligent patient will then ask, "How long has this operation been being done?"—a query to determine adequacy of follow-up. Even

---

*"Vitapulp," Pelston and Crane, P.O. Box 3664, Charlotte, N.C. 28203.

though the reply is "for about 20 years," neither the patient nor you the surgeon should forget that two decades is a comparatively short time to establish without question the safety of a procedure such as augmentation mammoplasty in patients whose chances of having breast cancer will increase until the age of 80 to 89. Presumably, the surgeon will not augment a patient with markedly nodular breasts, with previous biopsies, and a strong family history of breast cancer (in a premenopausal mother, sister, maternal aunt, and maternal grandmother).

Patients should be told that their gel prosthesis, especially if placed above the pectoral muscle, may make subsequent examination of the breasts difficult for some doctors and may cause x-ray films and xeroradiograms to be harder to read. Your responsibility is to be sure this patient understands that periodic self-examination and visits to the doctor are essential. Once so preoccupied by her breasts, she may now refuse to think about them in terms of their malignant potential. Unlike the padded bra breast, the implanted breast is now real, her own, well incorporated into her body image.

CLOSED CAPSULOTOMY.   Most plastic surgeons do not charge their own patients for closed capsulotomy following augmentation mammoplasty. However, for patients of a colleague, I usually charge a modest fee unless the surgeon has specifically requested otherwise. Capsulotomy in the office may seem simple but occasionally there are complications: hematoma, rupture of the implant, or asymmetry from a differential splitting of the scar tissue around both breasts. Now the breasts, though softer, may match less well. You should inform patients of all these possibilities. Also beware of giving intravenous medication, such as diazepam (Valium), in the office to ease the pain unless you are prepared to treat cardiac and pulmonary arrest.

INSTRUCTIONS.   The patient must know precisely your postoperative regimen: activity (at home, at work, athletics, sex), whether to change the dressings, when to begin breast massage, if you advise this. Some surgeons have observed that patients may be reluctant to massage their breasts because of fear of rupturing or dislodging the implant and because they are shy about what they might feel is a form of masturbation.

Many patients ask specifically whether the implant can rupture and the answer is "yes, but only very rarely." The usual question is "Will it rupture if I am in an auto accident?" I say that it probably will not but if it did, it likely would have saved her life by protecting her from severe thoracic injury.

Correction of Gynecomastia
This operation is one of the few cosmetic procedures sought exclusively by men.

PATIENTS
Usually in their teens or early 20s, patients for correction of gynecomastia are acutely embarrassed by the feminine appearance of their chest. In an effort to rid themselves of the stigma, they have done thousands of push-ups and hoisted tons of steel. The unfortunate result is a hypertrophy of their pectoral muscles and an increase in their mammary projection.

In your history taking, it is important to find out whether the patient has received testosterone injections for associated hypogonadism. I have had two such patients in whom occult cancer was found in their resected breast tissue.

Unlike patients for rhinoplasty, who are frequently accompanied by both parents, these patients, if adolescents, usually come with only one parent, the one more sympathetic to their problem. Often, these patients and their families have never been informed of the possibility of surgery; rather, the boy has been told that his gynecomastia will disappear when he is older and if he loses weight. The patient with adiposogenital dystrophy (Frölich's syndrome), or simply the "fat kid," may never grow out of his problem. Subjected to a multitude of laboratory tests, endocrinological evaluations, and testicular examinations, he looks upon surgery as a relief and once he knows that he can have it, he wants it as soon as possible. He does not wish to suffer through another summer, avoiding the beaches, making awkward excuses for not going swimming or for wearing his T-shirt on a scorching August day.

There may be a family history of gynecomastia but uncovering this information may embarrass the father, if present.

PHYSICAL EXAMINATION

You should examine the breasts carefully for discrete masses. Check the axillae for palpable nodes and the abdomen for an enlarged liver. Does the patient have a normal male escutcheon and are both testicles present and normal? (Hopefully, this will be the patient's last genital exam in relation to gynecomastia.)

Be certain to distinguish the patients who have only apparent gynecomastia; their problem may be simply hypertrophy of the nipple. Obviously, a more minor procedure is indicated for this problem than for the usual gynecomastia.

INFORMING THE PATIENT

Most cases of gynecomastia require essentially a bilateral subcutaneous mastectomy. This is usually done through an intraareolar incision. The patient must realize that he will have scars, usually not noticeable unless his gynecomastia is formidable. The operation then may necessitate incisions beyond the areola, small flaps of breast with the areola-nipple complex, grafts of the nipple and areola, or an extensive circumareolar approach.

The main complication with the usual operation for gynecomastia is postoperative bleeding, despite careful hemostasis. Seromas following removal of the drains (suction) even after four to five days can occur, and although not serious, are annoying. Also, the patient who notices the swelling may be very anxious because he fears that he will still have the same problem despite your reassurance otherwise.

Infection, although always a possibility, is unusual.

Changes in sensation do occur but only one patient, who was married, said it was disturbing because his nipples had long been a focus of pleasure for him and his wife. In a year, sufficient sensation returned to allow them to resume their usual activity but even after two years, the sensation was less than it had been before operation.

Although you may be justifiably concerned about causing a concavity from excessive removal of tissue, the patient will object more to a convexity from an insufficient procedure. I recall a 19-year-old whom the resident told that I would do the procedure very carefully so that there would be no noticeable indentation. When I later saw the patient, he was very worried that I would do less than he wished. "I don't care if I get a hollow there," he said, "just get all of it out. I don't want to go around with these [breasts] anymore."

PAYMENT

In almost every instance, correction of gynecomastia is cosmetic. An admitting diagnosis such as *mass of the breast(s)* or an operating title such as *mastectomy* is usually a ruse to obtain third-party coverage. This practice does little to enhance the status or reputation of medicine in general or the doctor in particular. Aside from such lofty considerations, not telling the truth by falsifying insurance forms is fraudulent and illegal.

AFTER OPERATION

You will relieve the anxiety of most patients by telling them immediately prior to operation that when they awake they will have bulky dressings. If you do not mention this, they will be extremely upset by their chest appearing even larger than it was before surgery.

Unless there are complications, patients stay in the hospital for just two days. Their drains can be removed in your office.

You must tell the patient how much and what sort of physical activity he is allowed. It is a rare patient who does not ask you repeatedly whether the swelling "will ever go down." These patients must be seen and reassured frequently because of their concern that you did not "take enough out."

For a comparatively simple operation, you will have generally a most grateful patient if you do not make the mistake of doing too little.

Correction of Breast Asymmetry or Agenesis

Unilateral or bilateral agenesis of the breast or marked asymmetry is usually very distressing psychologically to the female so affected. Many patients say that they have been ashamed of their condition to the degree that they have kept it a secret from their parents, siblings, and friends. Some girls may have told their mothers about their problem but have not allowed them to see it.

Since those who seek plastic surgery have obviously not adjusted to their abnormality, they may not be representative of all those with mammary agenesis or asymmetry. But many whom I have treated have shown extremes in their heterosexual behavior: avoidance of contact with men or promiscuity, the latter seemingly to prove to themselves that they can still be women despite their abnormality. Illegitimate pregnancies and abortions are also common—again a reaffirmation of their feminine capability. One patient with almost total absence of one breast said to me, "I couldn't wait to finish high school so I could marry and have children and nurse them." Pointing to her deficient breast, she announced proudly, "What a great surprise to see milk come out of that little thing."

Like the husbands of patients for augmentation or reduction, the spouse of a woman with mammary agenesis or asymmetry does not think that his wife has to undergo the surgery since he is not turned off sexually by his wife's anatomical problem. With a few patients, my impression was that the husband not only tolerated the deformity but liked it; not just in a sexual way but because he felt secure about having a wife who was insecure about her physical abnormality. These women's quest for reconstruction represents a step toward maturity and independence and may cause evident marital strain—whose ramifications for one patient and her husband led them to psychotherapy after she had had the operation; fortunately, the outcome was successful, anatomically and psychologically.

In your history taking, therefore, do not focus exclusively on the breast problem but attempt to understand its emotional meaning to the patient and those close to her.

PHYSICAL EXAMINATION
You must look carefully for abnormalities of the chest wall, pectoral musculature, and spinal column (scoliosis). Compare the breasts as to relative location, volume, shape, areolae, nipples. Ob-

serve what type (and size) of bra the patient is wearing. Does she use a prosthesis?

With asymmetry, always ask the patient which breast, if any, she likes. Occasionally, the patient may want the larger reduced; or the smaller augmented, or something done to each.

Many patients want either their mother or husband present during the examination. This helps to ensure that all concerned will know your findings and surgical plans. Sometimes the presence of someone else in the room, even a female nurse, is very upsetting to the patient. Be sensitive enough to recognize these differences and preferences. It does no harm to ask directly, "Stephanie, would you want your mother to be present when I examine you or would you prefer to have us discuss things with her afterwards?"

INFORMING THE PATIENT

By this time in the consultation, you should know what must be done: reduce or augment or both, inflatable or gel prosthesis or moulage or a combination. Remember that what you think is not the sole consideration. Make certain that you know what the patient wants. Is it possible to achieve it? If not, tell her. Spend time also to emphasize the impossibility of reconstructing a breast to match precisely the opposite. Stress that the operation will give improvement, hopefully, but never perfection. As with augmentation mammoplasty, the patient and family must understand the possibility of infection, hematoma, abnormal contour, and firmness. Indicate where you will make the incisions and what the expected scars will be.

BEFORE OPERATION

Many patients feel sufficiently embarrassed by their problem that they may prefer a private room and be willing to pay for it. In my experience, third-party payment is not usual for the correction of mammary agenesis or asymmetry.

AFTER OPERATION

In addition to your usual care of any patient or those after breast surgery, be especially attentive to the psychological reactions of these patients. Usually they are very happy with the improvement. However, an occasional patient may find readjustment difficult. Previously, her breast deformity was the reason (she told herself) for her avoiding normal social contact. Now she no longer has that excuse. It may be many months before she is willing to expose herself to a man. Be careful that you do not browbeat her with questions about this aspect of her life. She will feel more overwhelmed and inadequate. Most patients will let you know subtly or even openly that they have crossed the Rubicon.

Mastopexy

A pure mastopexy is a facelift of the breasts. It is an entirely cosmetic procedure and the patient will judge her result by esthetic standards.

PATIENTS

Patients for mastopexy are usually in their 30s and 40s and are white and middle class. The majority have had children and many attribute their sagging breasts to pregnancy and/or nursing. Another commonly invoked cause is rapid, significant weight loss. Patients say that the wilted appearance of the breasts depresses them. A common remark is, "I am only 40 but my breasts look like those of a 60-year-old." They may ask to have their breasts restored to what they once were—a size B or C. By that remark, they have introduced another aspect and that is breast volume. In taking the history, the plastic surgeon must determine whether the patient wishes not only to have her breasts raised but to have them enlarged. As with the patient for augmentation, these women seek the operation for themselves; the man in their life is usually perplexed by their persistent unhappiness with their breasts.

A thorough history should include information about general health, previous breast problems, if any, and familial predisposition to mammary malignancy.

PHYSICAL EXAMINATION

The surgeon must now assess whether the patient's problem is ptosis, and if so, whether it is severe enough to warrant an operation. In some patients, the condition is so mild that the scars for its correction would surely disturb them more than their ptosis.

It is important also to establish whether the patient needs not only a breast lift but also a reduction or augmentation. By raising the breasts with tension on the skin (your fingers or adhesive tape), you can let the patient judge whether the volume of the elevated breasts satisfies her. The breasts may be atrophic or hypertrophic as well as ptotic.

Your examination is not only to determine the type of procedure that will give the best appearance; careful palpation for possible masses is mandatory. These women generally are older and the possibility of breast cancer is not remote.

INFORMING THE PATIENT

This discussion with the patient must necessarily concern what is to be done: nothing, a mastopexy alone, or a mastopexy in conjunction with an augmentation or a reduction.

The patient must understand that any operation will leave permanent scars, even when the procedure is performed by a circumareolar incision whose resultant scar frequently widens. Do not underestimate this reality.

The principal decision usually for you and the patient is whether to do an augmentation. Adding a prosthesis to a markedly atrophic and ptotic breast without correcting the sagging will give a grotesque result. When a mastopexy and an augmentation are needed, the patient must understand that she may be subject to all the problems of both procedures but in particular those of the augmentation, especially abnormal firmness and abnormal contour. Many patients whose breasts are mildly or even moderately atrophic may elect to have only a mastopexy rather than run the risk of artificiality from a firm, unnatural breast. Many women worry that the presence of the prosthesis will interfere with subsequent breast examination and radiographic analysis—not an unreasonable fear. In my experience, doing the mastopexy first and the augmentation later is cumbersome planning; it makes the patient go through the operation twice, it increases cost and anxiety, and it does not produce a better result than the single-stage mastopexy/augmentation.

Some patients who describe their problem as sagging breasts actually have large, pendulous breasts that require a reduction. A few will ask to preserve the volume but raise the breasts. I remember well one woman to whose wish I grudgingly acceded. The result was a bulky breast whose areola and nipple projected displeasingly, pushed out by the excessive tissue. She later required the removal of breast parenchyma under the areola.

Patients for mastopexy alone must be told about possible changes in sensation, particularly around the nipple and areola, although in my experience these have been negligible, much less than after augmentation or reduction.

The major focus for discussion is to inform the patient that her scars will be permanent but the lift will probably not be: Time and gravity are likely to lower what you have so carefully raised. Most patients will ask how long the effects of the procedure last. You must honestly reply that you do not know since individuals vary in their wound healing, skin elasticity, genetic predisposition to aging of tissue; future health such as illnesses or pregnancy (with or without nursing); and weight fluctuation. You can point out that a sagging breast is somewhat like a sagging face; another surgical correction may be necessary. Since most patients know about repeat facelifts, they will better comprehend the problem through this simile.

For most women having mastopexy with or without augmentation, it can be done under local anesthesia with intravenous supplementation, on an outpatient basis. Some patients, particularly those requiring reduction, will do better with general anesthesia and a one- or two-day hospitalization, for which most will have insurance coverage only if the reduction is of sufficient magnitude to be considered functional. A scanty removal of skin and breast tissue does not justify calling the operation a reduction mammoplasty in order to obtain third-party payment. Insurance companies are right in being wary of these shenanigans.

AFTER OPERATION

As with every procedure, information to the patient must be clear and complete. With mastopexy, wearing a bra constantly for many weeks would seem advisable although as far as I know, there has been no objective study of the value of the bra in these circumstances. When an augmentation has been done in combination with the mastopexy, the dilemma is that you wish to free the patient from constricted dressings and to begin massage to keep things loose, an objective at cross-purposes to maintaining tightness of the repair.

Finally, all women must have periodic breast examination by a physician in addition to self-examination in order to detect any malignancy. After a year, the breast, if not augmented, will become soft; the more deeply placed scar tissue will not interfere with palpation. In patients 35 or older, baseline mammograms are helpful to serve as comparison should a future nodule be detected. In that circumstance, when the patient is beyond the immediate postoperative period, never hesitate to do a biopsy. Procrastination and false attribution of the nodule to "a stitch" or "scar tissue" could be disastrous.

Reduction Mammoplasty

This operation, which is being performed with increasing frequency, combines features of both esthetic and nonesthetic surgery. While there may be controversy about how to classify reduction mammoplasty, few would contest the observation that most patients are pleased with the results of their operation. Indeed, the more severe the macromastia, usually the happier the patient postoperatively unless a complication has occurred. Recently, however, as this procedure has become more popular, patients come with lesser degrees of hypertrophy. Some are in your office not primarily for a breast reduction but for a correction of ptosis. They may exaggerate their physical complaints—neck and back pain—in the hope of securing insurance coverage. For the surgeon, the difficulty is that they might judge the results by standards of appearance rather than by those of a function. One might comment sententiously that any good surgeon should be prepared to have his or her work appraised by "cosmetic" criteria. This type of patient, however, might become upset by minimal scarring, whereas another person requiring a significant breast reduction might be indifferent to the scars.

The age of patients wanting this surgery ranges from adolescent to postmenopausal. The older the woman or any patient, usually the more information you must know or will extract. Most women with very large breasts consider their condition a deformity. They feel conspicuous and resent being singled out for this aspect of themselves. They will complain that men fixate on their breasts to the exclusion of their personality or intellect [42]. Buying clothes is a frustrating and expensive experience. Unlike patients with small breasts who can hide their problem with a padded bra, patients with very large breasts, even with the most ingenious brassieres, still remain an object of scrutiny.

A common story is that patients will avoid athletics or going to the beach in a bathing suit. One woman said, "I dread each summer." In addition to these psychological problems, their macromastia may have had physical consequences: pain in the back, neck, and shoulder-strap areas, kyphosis, intertrigo, and obesity. Some patients consciously or unconsciously gain great amounts of weight, perhaps in an effort to make their breasts seem smaller in comparison. A psychiatrist who referred an 18-year-old girl for breast reduction told me that her obesity was a way of repulsing men to avoid an intimacy that would lead to exposure of her breasts. This low self-esteem is a frequent finding in patients with severely enlarged breasts.

Many patients will describe futile consultations with male pediatricians and family doctors who never suggested that surgery was possible, or warned them against it, or advised them to adapt to their large breasts because later men would like them. They have become long-suffering victims of male ignorance and chauvinism.

Often the younger patient is accompanied by her mother, who has also had to bear this problem without relief. The father is usually not present because he is "completely opposed," as the mother usually says, to the procedure. At best, fathers agree to the operation only with great reluctance.

PHYSICAL EXAMINATION
The surgeon who treats the female breast is dealing not only with an organ of appearance and function but with one subject to carcinogenesis. He or she should always be aware that the patient could have or could develop a carcinoma and every means must be taken to rule out its presence. Remember that the outer quadrant is

the most common location for carcinoma. A systematic breast examination should include palpating for cervical, axillary, and supraclavicular nodes, the last being an often neglected but frequent site of metastasis from primary breast cancer. Because of the large size of the breasts, physical examination is difficult but should nevertheless be performed thoroughly. Each breast should be inspected with the patient's arms at her sides, elevated, and behind her head—with the patient sitting and supine. Look for skin dimpling, surface flattening, nipple pointing (toward an adjacent tumor).

To detect curvature of the spine, the patient should be instructed to bend forward and to flex laterally while you are standing behind.

Note grooving and irritation of the shoulders from brassiere strap pressure. Sometimes, there is a decrease in sensation and motor power in the ulnar nerve distribution of the hand.

With the patient disrobed (and a nurse or family member present) I outline the incisions for the surgery. I then take photographs: front, side, oblique, and back.

Empathizing with the undressed patient, I suggest that she put on her clothes and then we can discuss the procedure more fully and with her more comfortable. The patient and the family must understand that reduction mammoplasty is major; it usually involves general anesthesia with approximately three to four hours of surgery, moderate pain, a two- to four-day hospitalization, and definite scarring. In addition, there is a possibility of infection (unusual), hematoma (uncommon), and ischemic necrosis of the nipple-areola complex as well as of the skin. No matter what the technique, there is always a chance of partial or total loss of the nipple and areola. The fact that you have done an operation 95 times without this occurrence does not mean that it will not happen later. Statistically, ischemic necrosis of the nipple-areola has an incidence of one to five percent, depending upon the series of patients reported. When you use the term "loss of the nipple" with the patient, you must explain it since she may think that you have simply mislaid it. The greater the weight of the tissue to be removed, the more frequent the complications.

Until recently, there was little appreciation of the fact that patients have altered sensation in the nipples, areolae, and breasts following reduction mammoplasty [29]. Preoperatively, the sensitivity of some patients with considerable hypertrophy is less than normal and postoperatively, their tactile sensitivity may improve. In the majority of instances, the sensation after surgery will be less. I have at least four patients in each of whom appreciation of touch has not returned to one nipple and areola after three years. I tell patients that for erotic purposes, they will have usually adequate sensation in their nipple and areola. Although objectively their appreciation of touch may be diminished, because they will feel better about themselves, they will be more relaxed during sex. It is important to speak openly and directly about these issues. Many patients will be too shy to raise the subject.

The surgeon must know the patient's expectations regarding size and shape. Although most women in my practice want to be a size B, some may specify an A and others a "good C." In this connection, discussing the procedure with the man in that patient's life is wise. Some men will sit in your office with obvious sullenness and hostility, angry that they will lose one (or two) of their prized possessions. To squire a woman with large breasts in our culture enhances the self-esteem of most men. Talking to the unhappy man before the operation may be helpful to avoid being in the middle or the focus of a squabble after surgery. I have had a few patients who have complained that their husband or boyfriend "has not come near me since the operation." Unconsciously or consciously, the man is retaliating in a passive-aggressive fashion. Occasionally, this situation has required a psychotherapist. A few women relate that the scars repel their partners. Often this obstacle can be overcome by suggesting to the patient that she wear her bra during intercourse for a few times.

OBESITY

The obese patient is generally more likely to have a complication than the individual of normal weight. Ideally, it makes sense to wait until the patient has lost all or most of the weight she intends to shed before modifying her profile. However, in my experience, the breast reduction provides the best stimulus for weight reduction. Many patients feel that whatever they do to lose weight will make little difference so long as they have large, unwieldy, and unsightly breasts. Furthermore, this deformity acts as a barrier to their exercising, especially in public.

AUTOTRANSFUSION

Although most patients undergoing reduction mammoplasty will not require blood transfusion, a few will. It is sometimes difficult to predict these patients but it is wise to check for anemia prior to scheduling them. The surgeon who believes that a transfusion is likely should make arrangements for the patient herself to give blood within three weeks of her operation. Daily oral iron supplements preoperatively and for three weeks postoperatively will help restore her blood cell volume. The patient will thus receive blood with almost no risk of hepatitis. Another method of decreasing the need for transfusion is, of course, the use of epinephrine at the time of surgery.

INSURANCE COVERAGE

This operation is generally covered by most insurance plans. However, the patient who has maximum ptosis but little hypertrophy may have difficulty in obtaining third-party payment. Justifiably, the insurance company will consider the procedure cosmetic, not functional. As mentioned, the patient will also judge the procedure in esthetic terms.

MAMMOGRAMS

In every patient 35 or older, I obtain mammograms. Since the breasts of these patients are particularly hard to examine, mammograms might be more helpful in them than in patients with normal sized breasts. In over 17 years of practice, I must admit that I have yet to detect a malignancy by this technique.

About a year after surgery, I again obtain mammograms, which then serve as a baseline for possible future detection of a breast abnormality.

AFTER OPERATION

Although ultimately most patients having had reduction mammoplasty will be satisfied with the result, not every woman immediately after operation is ecstatic. It is important that you do the first dressing change. Despite the considerable discussion that you may have had with the patient about ultimate breast size, she may react to her new look with surprise, dismay, and even denial. Some patients will declare, "I don't even want to look at them." Usually, however, they do sneak a glance and are pleased or unhappy. Few are indifferent. Some actually become weak and dizzy. Some say, "They don't look like mine and they don't feel like mine." Or, "Will they ever look like breasts?"

You had expected gratitude for relieving her of deforming burdens; now perplexed and disappointed, you stand uneasily at the bedside. Before you become angry and stomp out of the room, remember that she has to make a major adjustment in her body image. Unlike the patient after a facelift who remembers when she was young, the big-breasted patient, especially if middle-aged or older, may never recall having a normal bosom. Moreover, if she is obese, her breasts following reduction may appear especially small compared to the rest of her. If she had intended to lose weight, gently remind her that you have gauged her surgery to match what she will look like (if that is what you truly did). Your statement to her brings to mind the exchange between Pablo Picasso and Gertrude Stein, who said, after she saw his portrait of her, "It does not look like me," to which Picasso replied, "It will."

Reassure the patient that her feelings of bewilderment and depression are not unusual but ordinarily pass in several weeks after she becomes more accustomed to her new breasts and body contour. Psychological adjustment only occasionally requires psychiatric help if she has your support and availability as well as an understanding family and friends, especially the male members. You can do much before operation and afterward to prepare her intimates to deal with these new problems of adaptation.

Following removal of the drains (on the second postoperative day), I usually send the patient home in a bra (Sears Catalogue #78495, cup C–D). The patient is responsible for her dressing changes, which should be done by herself preferably or by a friend or a member of the family. I usually advise patients to wear a bra day and night for four to six weeks. With normal healing, she can resume driving and sex at a week and athletics between two and three weeks after surgery.

As doctors, we have a responsibility to the patient beyond the immediate operation. The fact that someone has had a reduction mammoplasty does not confer immunity from breast cancer. Any suspicious lump should be biopsied and not simply ascribed to "scar tissue" or "stitch reaction." Many patients request that you periodically examine their breasts because "My doctor says he is not used to checking breasts that have had this kind of surgery."

Aside from the oncological value of doing the breast examination, long-term follow-up will give you important information about your results. You will then be better able to evaluate the technique you used and you will be more knowledgeable when informing patients about what they can expect from this operation. Frequently the patient is more pleased than you. You will note unattractive scarring, slight asymmetry, unwanted fullness, elevated nipple, or altered sensation. Resist the temptation to proclaim, "Mea culpa." Expressing your dissatisfaction may make you feel more honest but will also make the patient more unhappy. Being a good physician also requires knowing when to remain silent. Inwardly record your observations so that you may do a better procedure for the next patient. But remember also that variations in technique will not necessarily give a perfect result.

Reconstruction After Mastectomy

Grudgingly but gradually, the medical profession has recognized the needs and rights of women for reconstruction after mastectomy. The preponderance of men in medicine accounted for the negative attitude that breast reconstruction was frivolous. Consciously or unconsciously, their concept was that breasts are an adornment, something once there for species preservation but now present for male pleasure. This chauvinistic stance is far from what breasts mean to a woman. Notman [105], a psychiatrist and a woman, has written,

> For a woman they [breasts] represent an important component of her femininity, combining nutrient maternal potential with sexual attractiveness. Her capacity to nourish and to give is important not only in her actual functions as a nursing mother or in the role of a lover, but in creating the sense of worthwhileness and adequacy which underlies self-

esteem . . . . The significance of her breasts to a woman goes beyond realistic considerations alone . . . the symbolic importance of the breasts remains throughout life.

Since breast cancer is occurring in younger women but its incidence increases with every decade until 80 to 89, patients having had a mastectomy and wanting breast reconstruction range widely in age. In my series, the youngest has been 19, the oldest, 72.

Not every woman who has had a breast removed wants a reconstruction. But almost every patient having had a mastectomy must deal with the threat to her life, the physical, emotional, and interpersonal responses to trauma and crisis, her fear about the loss and the mutilation, her concern about her sexual attractiveness, her anxiety about recurrent cancer or new cancer in the opposite breast, and her dread of confronting her own disfigurement. In addition, women after mastectomy have practical problems such as buying and wearing clothes and being in a bathing suit. Their freedom is constrained [123]. They frequently say, "I can never be just in a housedress at home. If anyone comes to the door, he will see that I am lopsided." External prostheses are cumbersome; they slip and macerate the skin. Furthermore, the woman never internalizes them since, in reality, they are not internal. Putting on the special bra and prosthesis in the morning becomes a despised ritual. It these women have asked themselves, "Why me?" with regard to their cancer, they now query, "Why not me?" with respect to reconstruction. For many women, the impasse to having a breast made is not their psyche but that of their surgeon, who did the mastectomy but is opposed to reconstruction. His or her reasons may be medical but often they are puritanical and punitive: Restoring a breast is self-indulgence and vanity; the patient is lucky to be alive and she should not complain about a minor matter. Unconsciously, the male surgeon may feel that the patient should pay for her survival with suffering. Fortunately, with the pressures from the press and the media and the experiences of other patients, and the increasing number of younger sympathetic surgeons, many of whom are women, women are finding more support in their quest to be whole again. The male surgeon should realize that the patient wants the reconstruction for herself, not to please a sexual partner. The usual story for the patient is that she desires the reconstruction but her husband is opposed to it because he thinks it is unnecessary, he is afraid of the risks, and he does not want his wife to go through more pain and hospitalization. Many women frankly admit that their husbands want to have sex with them but they, even in a bra, feel "deformed" or "freakish" and back away. That the reconstruction of the breast is a family affair is evidenced by the usual presence of the husband or fiancé. Often the woman has been so depressed by the mastectomy with its many implications that she has ceased to function adequately as a mother and wife. In these circumstances, the family are urging reconstruction in the hope that it will lift the iron veil from their home. In seeing the interaction between husband and wife and his concern for his wife's physical and emotional well-being, one realizes the need of human beings for each other and one also has an inkling of how difficult the adjustment may be for the isolated female.

HISTORY

In taking the history, you should know the precise diagnosis and operation (you may have to request the other surgeon's records), whether the axillary nodes were positive, and whether the patient has had irradiation or chemotherapy or both.

Inquire also about family history since this information may determine the management of the opposite breast. In your focus on the breast, do not neglect the rest of the body: allergies, previous operations, cardiovascular and pulmonary status, current medications, smoking history.

PHYSICAL EXAMINATION

Your examination should tell you about presence or absence of recurrent disease, the state of the scars and soft tissue (thick, atrophic, mobile, fixed), the presence or absence of the pectoral muscles. In addition, you should appraise the opposite breast. Notice configuration. Will it be difficult to match the reconstructed side to it? Since the chance of malignancy developing at some time in the opposite breast is about 10 percent, examine it carefully. Also palpate for axillary nodes bilaterally. Is there lymphedema in the arm?

Make note of the patient's body proportions, which are relevant to the reconstruction.

While the patient is undressed, take this opportunity to photograph her and to explain how you plan to do the reconstruction. You can also measure the volume of the operative breast (Breast Measurement Device—Krianoff Design)* and the size of the patient's prosthesis, if not porous, by water displacement.

INFORMING THE PATIENT

Before I outline steps toward a reconstruction, I emphasize that I shall communicate with her surgeon and family doctor. When they have referred the patient, the situation is much easier than if either or both are opposed to the reconstruction. In that instance, I send a letter describing the patient's desire for reconstruction and how it would be done. Often I state openly that the patient said "you are opposed to the idea but we both hope that you will reconsider your position in view of what it means to her and what it has meant to other patients with similar problems." In your conversation with the patient and in your letter to her doctors, you should mention that you have asked her to consult them after they have received the letter. A copy to the patient is helpful; indicate on your original that you have sent her one.

Sometimes, reconstruction must be delayed because the patient is uncertain about whether she wishes it or because it is too soon after mastectomy or because she is receiving irradiation or chemotherapy or both.

If the patient is prepared to have the procedure and her physicians are in agreement, I take the patient through the steps of the operation: a hospitalization of two to three days, general anesthesia for an operation that takes about an hour and a half (unless a musculocutaneous flap is to be used), the expected pain (moderate), and her going home in a bra and resuming work in approximately seven to ten days after operation. I recommend no driving for a week and no tennis or golf for about three weeks. Whatever your regimen, this is the time to outline it to the patient, who must arrange for coverage at work and in her home.

---

*McGhan Medical Corporation, 700 Ward Drive, Santa Barbara, Calif. 93111.

Patients should know about the possibilities of infection and hematoma (both uncommon) and asymmetry. They should understand they could lose the prosthesis through extrusion, perhaps as a result of ischemic necrosis of the skin or infection.

A major decision is the management of the opposite breast: to leave it alone, reduce it, perform subcutaneous of simple mastectomy. Your advice in this matter must be individualized. Perhaps a worrisome previous biopsy or family history will lead you to recommend a simple or a subcutaneous mastectomy. This is not the place to list the advantages and disadvantages of these different methods.

Some patients would rather leave a large pendulous breast intact despite the marked asymmetry because their wish to have "one normal breast" or, as one patient expressed it, "one breast that is my own and that has not had you surgeons at it." The decision about the opposite breast should be made in consultation with the patient's surgeon. If a biopsy has been done, you should obtain the slides and view them with your pathologist. Sometimes the general surgeon (the gynecologist) prefers to leave the opposite breast unscarred in order to be able to examine it more effectively clinically and radiographically. As you discuss the different approaches, you will get an idea of what the patient and her husband prefer. Frequently, the patient appears bewildered by the many choices. The reality, I tell them, is, "It is not a black and white matter. You have different alternatives and I want to give you the benefit of all the pros and cons, even at the expense of confusing you initially." With some patients, a return visit is helpful. She will have had more time to think about the problem and the alternatives, and will have talked with her surgeon and family physician. Another consideration is whether and when to reconstruct the nipple and areola. I usually do this at a second stage, on an outpatient basis, approximately three months after the breast reconstruction. I can then site the nipple with more precision. In my practice, only 2 of 10 women actually have it done. The others seem satisfied with just the breast mound.

The various methods of nipple-areola reconstruction have their advantages and disadvantages. The patient should be informed about them without wearying her with details. One woman whose nipple I reconstructed with a cartilage graft from the ear called my attention to a disadvantage of that technique: The nipple is always erectile, unlike its normal opposite. This difference can be embarrassing and noticeable if the patient wears a tightly fitting sweater or blouse. If you are contemplating using a latissimus dorsi flap or something similar, you must discuss the procedure with the patient. Here slides are helpful to describe the method and results since the technique may confuse the patient and the family. Mention the possibility of flap failure even though the probability may be small. Also make certain that the patient and the family understand that after elevating the flap, it is not always possibile to transfer it if there is indication of insufficient blood supply. The patient who is expecting a transfer of the flap will be justifiably disappointed and angry if she has not been forewarned of that small likelihood that another stage will be necessary.

The media have made the public aware of breast reconstruction, and this may account for that patient's being in your office. However, because many articles in the press have exaggerated the esthetic result of the surgery, the patient and her family may have unrealistic expectations. Those patients are the only group to whom I routinely show photographs of *average* results as well as of certain unfavorable outcomes, such as capsular contracture and asymmetry. In this regard, I tell the patient and her family that she will look better in a bra and I have photographs that illustrate this fact. The purpose of the pictures is not to sell the operation but to document graphically its limitations so that the patient will not be dissatisfied afterward.

Although the patient's satisfaction with the result usually exceeds the actual anatomical attainments, not every woman will be pleased and grateful with your best. To paraphrase Sam Goldwyn, "Include them out" at your initial consultation.

AFTER OPERATION

The first dressing change may be a pleasant or unpleasant experience for the patient. Generally, with time, the reconstructed breast projects more than it does initially, when its shape is amorphous. The patient must be reassured about this and that is why your presence will be valuable support to her. It is wise to instruct those close to her, such as her husband and friend(s), to support her emotionally during this early phase. You and they must urge her not to expect the final result within the first couple of weeks.

I remember one patient, a 48-year-old separated city planner, who became very depressed just after her reconstruction. I thought the reason was her dissatisfaction with the shortcomings of the procedure. In fact, she did say that she had expected "something more" than what she saw at the first dressing change. She did acknowledge, however, that she had "quite an improvement." A few days later in my office, she analyzed her emotional state as being due to "a reawakening of all the feelings I had at the time of my mastectomy four years ago." At my suggestion, she called the psychotherapist who had helped her then. With time and after talks with him by phone (she had moved from the Midwest) her mood returned to what it had been before operation.

There are patients who become depressed after any major surgical procedure; their reactive depression probably has a different etiology, perhaps biochemical, than that in the patient just described, who had gone through operations other than on her breast without subsequent depression.

As with any other procedure, the patient after breast reconstruction must know what she should do about dressing changes, exercising, driving, and housework. Sending the patient home in a brassiere helps immeasurably to restore her self-confidence. It is important also to give specific advice about when to resume sex, since this might be the ultimate test for the patient of the operation's success. Generally I suggest that after four or five days, intercourse is allowed, but "no weight on top for two weeks." My reason for being so specific is that I was once awakened in the middle of the night by a patient whom I had not instructed but who asked me, "Is it alright to go ahead now?"

Postoperative care includes continued vigilance for recurrent cancer or new malignancy in the opposite breast. The fact that the breast has been reconstructed has not eliminated that woman's cancer potential. Be certain that the patient is being adequately evaluated at regular intervals, preferably by her original surgeon and/or her oncologist as well as by you.

Abdominoplasty

Most patients for abdominoplasty are middle-aged women; men who seek the operation usually have lost a considerable amount of weight and cannot exercise away the remaining apron of skin and fat. The woman patient may have a lax abdomen because of a major weight loss but, more frequently, because of childbearing, with perhaps one or more caesarean sections. Slender patients commonly say, "I really hate myself in the summer. I want to wear a bikini." From such an expression, one might conclude that they are undertaking the surgery for a frivolous reason. Compared to submitting to coronary bypass, it may be. But a clue to their true motivation is not the last part of their statement—the desire to wear a bikini—but the first part, their negative feelings about themselves. To them their skin redundancy is disagreeable evidence of the effects of aging and mothering [70]. Instead of a badge of self-fulfillment, the crinkly skin has become a reminder of their body's decline. Many patients who have recently been divorced or widowed want to start a new life. Recently a widow remarked, "I wish that I were a snake so I could get new skin." Another patient, a divorcée, commented, "I feel like a used car when I see myself without clothes." What she might have said is that she felt like an *abused* car, since she thought that her husband had treated her badly and that she had given him and the children "her best years without any appreciation."

Because an abdominoplasty, even if minimal, involves hospitalization and general anesthesia, and approximately a three-hour operation, it certainly cannot be considered "minor," if, indeed, any operation ever is. Abdominoplasty demands a thorough past history and systems review. You should also inquire about the patient's plans for more pregnancies, an event that theoretically might worsen your surgical result.

If the patient is planning to have another child in the near future, it would be better to postpone the abdominoplasty.

PHYSICAL EXAMINATION

The purpose of your examination is to determine whether or not the patient will benefit from an abdominoplasty and, if so, to what extent.

How much skin laxity is there? Does he or she have a diastasis recti or a hernia? Does the patient want the operation as a shortcut to losing weight? Should the patient shed poundage before undertaking surgery?

There is a category of patients who even with a well-executed abdominoplasty will still look as if not much had been accomplished. They are pudgy with thick skin and fat, often with lordosis. They should lose weight and tighten their back and abdominal musculature before an accurate prognosis can be given about the benefits of abdominoplasty.

INFORMING THE PATIENT

Unfortunately, the public may consider abdominoplasty a "tummy tuck," and some plastic surgeons may reinforce this misconception by minimizing the extent of the surgery and the type and degree of complications [69]. The patient must be told and must understand that fatalities have occurred; that pulmonary embolism is a possibility, as are infection, hematoma, and loss of skin from ischemia and dehiscence. The incisions used should be explained again (the first time should be during the physical examination) and the patient must realize that the scars will be permanent, hopefully not prominent but possibly thick, red, and ugly. Do not neglect to mention the scars around the umbilicus. Do not forget also to discuss altered sensation of the abdominal wall. Occasionally, the patient may be bothered by numbness and paresthesias. Theoretically, there may be a difference in the localization of abdominal pain because of the shift of the abdominal wall tissues.

Patients must know the degree of expected improvement in abdominal contour. It is seldom more than they expect; it frequently is less. For example, unless an incision is made around the waist, the fatty, redundant lateral tissue will remain. Most surgeons do not do a torsoplasty because of the resultant scars, but the patient may expect to be transformed from the usual 40-year-old into a supple ballet dancer. In this regard, men generally have fewer expectations, overt or covert.

Female patients will usually ask whether the striae will disappear. The answer, of course, is "no," but they may be improved by the tightening.

Abdominoplasty involves more pain and discomfort and more time for complete resumption of all activities than does a rhinoplasty, for example. Patients, especially mothers, want to know when they can begin car pooling, baby lifting, shopping, and housework.

Since most insurance policies do not include this type of surgery, its cost must be borne by the patient. Do not underestimate the length of hospitalization and the charges for the operating room, the anesthesia, and the admission studies, including an electrocardiogram and chest x-ray films.

It is helpful to be able to discuss all these aspects with the patient's family—spouse, parent—or even a friend. The principal reason is to be certain that all concerned realize that an abdominoplasty is a serious venture.

Since abdominoplasty is often done along with other procedures, most commonly augmentation mammoplasty or correction of breast ptosis, the surgeon and the patient must decide how much should be planned for that particular day. Although doing more than one procedure in one session on a patient may be attractive from a time-cost point of view, it sometimes boomerangs to the disadvantage of both the patient and the surgeon. Occasionally the second procedure is not done so carefully as the first unless the surgeon is fast and unless there is another team available. This does not mean, however, that you should not schedule an abdominoplasty with, for example, augmentation mammoplasty, but you must know how much you and your patient can tolerate. Prepare the patient also for another possible postoperative discomfort: having an indwelling catheter for a couple of days. This can be an unpleasant surprise for a patient awakening from surgery who has not been informed. Notify the patient also of the flexed position of the hips after operation and explain its rationale.

Thigh and Buttocks Lift

Candidates for these operations are usually women. They are seeing you because they dislike the prominence of their hips and the sagging and bulkiness of their buttocks and thighs. These may be familial characteristics that have concerned them since adolescence. Perhaps with age, weight gain, or weight fluctuation, their tissues have become fatter, flabbier, and more ptotic. Male patients wanting this surgery have lost a considerable amount of weight and complain about the severely hanging skin.

In an effort to streamline themselves, most patients have made a fetish of exercising with an emphasis on cycling (and exercise bike) as much as 50 miles a day, with the result of adding more muscle to their thighs and buttocks but still not significantly reducing the sagging. Massage, "cellulite" treatment centers, slenderizing parlors, and friction belts may help some individuals but the patients in your office have tried them all without success and you are their last hope.

Many women with heavy thighs and buttocks never wear shorts. They dislike their thighs "rubbing together," assuming others think it is unattractive; it may also irritate their skin. They also may say that for many years their "secret desire" has been to get into a pair of jeans.

Some patients have excess tissue not only in their buttocks. Bernard Berenson [12] recounted the incident of a gloomy lady who was asked why she was sad. "How would you feel if, like me, you had to pass the rest of your days between a big bosom and a bigger behind?" For such people, a program of weight loss by diet should precede any consideration of weight loss by surgery.

Because a thigh and buttocks lift usually involves a hospitalization, general anesthesia, and three or more hours of surgery, you must inquire about the patient's past health, history of allergies, and current medications, if any. Compared to an eyelidplasty or a facelift or rhinoplasty, this surgery demands a longer recuperative period.

PHYSICAL EXAMINATION
The patient should indicate to you during the examination what bothers him or her. You can then determine whether the operation will meet expectations.

Depending upon the specific areas of concern, the degree of laxity of the skin, and the amount of fat, the problem of the thighs, for example, sometimes can be resolved by only a medial excision of tissue; other patients require a lateral approach as well, and still others are best served by no operation. In this last group are those who are squat, with thick, firm tissue and muscle and heavy bones. Since there is no sagging of tissue, there is little to lift. An operation will give that patient discomfort, expense, scars, and disappointment. Another type of patient from whom to stay your knife is the person whose complaint is the gathering of tissue at the knees, particularly medially. Surgery by the usual incisions in the inguinal and gluteal areas will cause only a mild improvement distally. A direct attack on the problem with a vertical medial incision is usually unwarranted unless there is an enormous amount of tissue to remove and even then, the resultant scars usually make this operation unacceptable to the patient as well as to the surgeon. Sometimes, a patient will notice the beginnings of aging and its consequent minimal sagging. In that situation, surgery will do little for him or her. By pinching and pulling on tissue at various sites in the buttocks and thighs, you can give a patient some idea of what the prospective operation can do.

Examine the patient carefully for scar potential by scrutinizing preexisting incisions. Ask also about possible family tendency to keloids.

INFORMING THE PATIENT

As mentioned, a thigh and/or buttocks lift is a major undertaking and the spectrum of possible complications includes dehiscence and death. Infection and hematoma may occur but the principal problems are the limitation in improvement and the permanence of scars. If only a modest (a euphemism for "negligible") benefit can be anticipated, I discourage the patient from surgery. Frequently scars will descend with time to a visible level even when you thought you had placed the incisions sufficiently high. Patients will then have to wear a longer bathing suit to cover your surgical tracks.

Patients having more than just a medial thighplasty should be told that they will walk stiffly for about two or three weeks because of pulling at the incisions. They will also have difficulty in dressing, climbing stairs, and getting in and out of bed. They should not expect to sit comfortably or to drive for seven to ten days or to play golf or tennis for about three weeks. To some patients who expect to get a noticeable improvement, these facts are not a deterrent.

In my practice and that of many others, the number of patients having thigh and/or buttocks lift has decreased, largely because the improvement is not always significant; the scars are real and lasting; and time and gravity can only lower what you have raised.

As with patients for abdominoplasty, you should inform them that they will be on urinary catheter drainage for a few days. If your preoperative and postoperative routine is a low–residue diet, notify them also about this.

Scar Revision

Some might argue that this procedure is not "cosmetic" but "reconstructive," "restorative," "rehabilitative." Whatever its cubbyhole, it is certain that the advent of seat belts and shatterproof glass in cars has significantly decreased the incidence of severe facial lacerations and the number of patients wanting revision of facial scars. The dog seems to have replaced the auto in causing scars of the face, particularly in children.

PATIENTS

The majority of patients for scar revision come at the instigation of an attorney or claims agent. Always in the background is the question of legal proceedings. Sometimes the scar(s) is so small that you think "only in America" could this stir such a tempest. Other patients, however, have such ugly scars that you wonder how they every adapted to their condition.

History taking should be precise, not only because it is better medicine but because you will probably have to send a letter to the patient's lawyer or insurance company. Frequently, the circumstances are unclear and the patient's reporting is biased. Record all that the patient says; do not attempt to unravel the skein, since that is the job of the attorneys or court. Inquire about previous treatment: when, where, by whom? Were there associated injuries, bony, visceral, cerebral? Was there subsequent infection in the repaired lacerations? What has been the interim management: steroid injection, massage with vitamin E or cocoa butter, further surgery? If the patient has had other consultations, it is helpful to obtain these reports in addition to the operating notes and hospital records.

The patient should be questioned specifically concerning the scars: physical or psychological pain, functional impairment, particularly with scars around the mouth and eyes or on the extremities. Answers to these questions may not always be honest because the patient or family or both are aware that the greater the complaint, the larger the financial settlement. Your business, however, is to record, not cross-examine.

Sometimes the patient is in your office because the insurance company has recommended an "impartial" consultation. The patient and the family may be accompanied by their lawyer and may consider you a hired hand, retained by the insurance company to give an opinion unfavorable to the patient. I always say that I do not work for any insurance company (the truth) but I have been asked to provide an objective evaluation, which I shall communicate in writing. I also make clear that I am not trying to displace another physician in the care of that patient. After these declarations, the wariness and hostility noticeably decrease.

PHYSICAL EXAMINATION

For your records, as well as for those of the attorney and insurance company, you should state the location of the scars and their appearance (color; whether raised or depressed, thick or thin), as well as their dimensions. Give a mirror to the patient, who can then indicate to you a scar that has faded well or one that is hidden, as on the scalp. At the same time, you can ask the patient whether the scars have improved and, if so, which ones? This will give you information about a scar that might be ready for revision.

By palpating the scars, you can judge their thickness and tenderness and, occasionally, you may find a foreign body, perhaps a piece of glass. In the face, it is important to record changes in sensation as well as the action of facial muscles, especially whether the frontalis is working normally. Some patients have a natural asymmetry of this muscle, unrelated to the accident. You should also palpate the facial bones for residual deformity if there has been a fracture. Occasionally, you may detect a fracture of which the patient is unaware.

With a child, you must rely on the observations of the parents. Sometimes, as mentioned, they may exaggerate the problems, perhaps because of their concern or desire for a more favorable recompense.

I usually do not send a report to the attorney until I receive payment since it is cumbersome to carry open accounts for the years that may pass before the case is concluded. You or your secretary may tell the patient that he or she can pay for the report and presumably the settlement will refund him or her, although there is no guarantee. Unlike law offices, insurance companies generally send an immediate payment as soon as you bill them and I do not ask, therefore, for prepayment.

In your letter to the attorney or insurance company, give as clearly and precisely as possible the history that you obtained and your findings on physical examination. Discuss also the patient's symptoms or lack of them: altered sensation, and emotional reactions to injury.

Make certain that you state that if a scar revision were to be done, you cannot guarantee the result but hopefully there will be an improvement. You might also declare that the scars are permanent insofar as you can judge at this time. With certain patients, you may have to withhold judgment because their injury is too recent and a better evaluation can be done in three to six months.

The attorney or insurance company will want to know what operation you might do and what it would cost. Again, you may have to defer such information until you are certain that the scar will benefit from revision. If you know that an operation is necessary, state your fee and the expected hospital costs. This is a good time also to mention that one or more operations might be necessary if that seems likely.

INFORMING THE PATIENT
Patients for scar revision may expect too much from that operation and they must understand, emotionally as well as intellectually, that you cannot eliminate a scar but hopefully may make it better. They should also realize that six months to a year must elapse before they will see the true results of your surgical inter-

vention. The patient and the family should know that scars in general, and scar revision in particular, have better outcomes in older persons than in adolescents. Parents usually have the misconception that the opposite is true. You must take the time to describe in detail your plans for scar revision. It is helpful for the patient to look at the scar in a mirror while you draw your lines for revision, such as a Z-plasty or W-plasty. Other myths to shatter are that we plastic surgeons do invisible mending and that we always use a skin graft or something plastic. Give the reasons a skin graft is usually not the best choice (looks forever like a patch), and stress again that once a scar, always a scar.

You should also discuss the circumstances under which you will do the scar revision. Most uncomplicated scars in adults and older children can be managed with local anesthesia on an outpatient basis. Occasionally, however, a patient, usually very young, may have been so upset emotionally by having been awake at the time of the original repair that he or she cannot tolerate the same conditions and may request and merit general anesthesia.

PATIENT PERMISSION FOR TRANSMITTAL OF INFORMATION
You must obtain the patient's permission in writing to send your report to the attorney, even when the attorney is the patient's. Once I inadvertently corresponded with the lawyer for the opposite party—an unfortunate gaffe! In the case of a minor, a parent or legal guardian must give permission.

THE QUESTION OF PAYMENT
Probably no area of surgery causes more confusion than scar revision with regard to payment. What I have found practical is a form that the patient or parent signs to affirm their responsibility to pay you no matter what the decision of the insurance company or the court. Lately, in fact, I have insisted on prepayment. If you do not do this, you will wait years before recovering your fee. When I was first in practice, I was more bashful and invariably regretted it. You can be a good doctor and still get paid. For the patient who is not financially able, you will make whatever arrangements you wish. For those in a university setting, having the patient become a resident's case and helping him do the surgery is

a good solution since the patient will then not be charged for your services and may have to pay only a minimal hospital bill, particularly if it is an outpatient procedure.

PHOTOGRAPHS
As with every patient, it is wise to take two sets of photographs. Almost certainly the attorney will ask for one, which you can furnish at a moderate fee.

WHEN TO OPERATE
This is not a textbook on plastic surgical care but many scars, even at six months, need maturing. Some scars are ready for revision much sooner than the usual three to six months' dictum. And, finally, some scars are better left alone, allowing time alone to do its scarless revision.

Beware of patients who have had a minimal scar for many years. They will probably expect more improvement than you can produce and will think that the red scar from the revision looks much worse than the old one that had many years to fade. Some patients with mild scarring will be surprised at your disclaimers—your refusal to guarantee a result. They will have heard about or even know someone who had "terrible scars" and had a plastic surgeon give them a "fantastic improvement." The point to emphasize is that it is easier to go from bad to good than from better to best. These are not simply semantic distinctions.

Dermabrasion of Acne Scars

The popularity of dermabrasion may exceed its value; the reason is lack of something better and the shared hope of patient and doctor that the result will justify its doing.

Most patients for dermabrasion have acne scars whose presence has bothered them emotionally for many years. Women may have had the benefit of makeup but they complain of the nuisance of applying it and the necessity of using many layers.

Almost every patient at some time has been under the care of a dermatologist; usually, but not always, the acne is no longer active. Today most patients have heard conflicting reports about the efficacy of dermabrasion and they are in your office to get information. They want to know whether the procedure will help them, how it would be done, whether it will be painful, and how much it will cost. Some patients, however, have already decided that they want dermabrasion and are seeing you to make definite arrangements.

For every patient, a thorough inquiry into general health, past illnesses, and allergies is necessary. Do not neglect to find out whether the patient had previous irradiation treatment and dermabrasion and with what results. Ask female patients whether they are taking oral contraceptives, since some types may produce hyperpigmentation after dermabrasion.

PHYSICAL EXAMINATION

With the patient holding a mirror, ask him or her to indicate which areas he or she would like improved. Usually it is both cheeks, perhaps the chin, maybe the forehead—sometimes all these areas. Occasionally, it is not an area that looks bad to you and it is wise to know this before you talk about treatment.

Note whether the patient has active acne. Frequently, the patient's skin looks unattractive not so much because of scarring but because of fresh acne eruptions.

INFORMING THE PATIENT

You must now decide how much you believe dermabrasion can improve the patient's condition. I usually tell a patient that "on a scale of 0 to 10 (10 being the most improvement), you will get a 3, 4, or 5," for example. The patient must understand that you are not filling in the scars but planing down the surrounding tissue—not building up the valleys but leveling the mountains. The patient must realize that dermabrasion does carry the danger of unwanted scarring, milia (explain what that is to the patient), and uneven pigmentation, usually increased in some areas—most often transient but occasionally permanent.

I tell patients that the most common unfavorable result is unhappiness from anticipating more improvement than is possible. Unfortunately, those patients with cystic acne scars need help the most but benefit the least. One patient, a male psychologist whom

I discouraged from the procedure, showed me a cartoon of Garfield in that morning's paper. A cat is saying, "Tomorrow I'll be two years of age. That's the human equivalent of fourteen . . . cats have it good. Adolescence without acne." For that patient, of course, for whom nothing could be done, the situation was not humorous.

For some patients in whom I am doubtful about the result, it is useful to select an area on the face to test dermabrade. This can easily be done in the office and the patch, about the size of a quarter, can then be observed for several months before deciding about further treatment. By this measure, the patient does not become committed, nor do I, to a larger, more expensive and unpredictable procedure perhaps without benefit.

Patients will usually ask about repeat dermabrasion—whether it is possible to do the procedure again should there be an improvement. The answer is that it can be done but it is usually better to see what the dermabrasion can accomplish before deciding on more treatment.

Since most patients do not have insurance coverage for dermabrading acne scars, they will have to pay the costs. This is true even when some pits have been excised in association with the dermabrasion.

Treatment of Port Wine Stains

Although only a few plastic surgeons presently use the argon laser for port wine stains, the number of potential patients is enormous. Since they and their families have had to cope with a noticeable congenital deformity, an analysis of their relationship to the plastic surgeon should be instructive.

PATIENTS

In my series, patients have ranged from infants to those in their late 60s. Older patients come because of their concern about their appearance; for those in infancy, the distress of the parents has prompted the consultation. Patients in their 50s or 60s may have been treated with dry ice, cauterization, sclerosing agents, irradiation, tattooing, or a combination of therapies. The younger the patient, the greater the likelihood that he or she has not had any medical or surgical attempt to improve the port wine stain since parents in the past two decades have been told that "nothing can be done." Camouflage by makeup is a standard recourse but is used more by women than by men.

The parents and the patient have usually heard or read something about the laser and generally their expectations are unrealistically high. Much of the time you spend with them is taken with stressing the limitations, the unpredictability, and the complications of the technique.

In taking the history, especially if the patient is an infant, you will soon realize that the mother, particularly, feels guilty that she has given birth to a child with a congenital deformity. For most patients, there is no family history of such a condition. Frequently, the mother and father will say that the child's grandparents have explained the appearance of the port wine stain by the mother's eating poorly during her pregnancy or having a fright, or doing something forbidden by superstition, such as eating raspberries or strawberries during the first trimester. As the parents relate these stories, they may smile nervously. They are obviously looking to you for reassurance that they did nothing wrong to cause their child's affliction. In general, the parents of the father are more accusing that those of the mother and the target is always the mother. Secretiveness, shame, guilt, and anger over a congenital abnormality are common and are seen flagrantly when the infant has been born with a cleft lip or cleft palate.

With any port wine stain of the face, especially involving the upper and lower lids, inquire about a recent ophthalmological examination to rule out the possibility of glaucoma, which is not uncommon with this condition.

INFORMING THE PATIENT AND FAMILY
Discussion with the patient and the family concerning the argon laser begins with a brief explanation of how the apparatus works and the theoretical explanation for its success. As mentioned, most of your consultation will center on possible unfavorable results of treatment. You must inform the patient (and family) about the

likelihood of failure, the possibility of hypertrophic scarring—
especially in patients younger than 17 and with a lighter port wine
stain—and the chance of a depressed scar at the site of treatment
[28]. A biopsy in conjunction with a test patch may provide helpful information to predict the patient's response to the argon laser
[103].

In addition to the verbal information, giving the patient a book-
let about the method is helpful. I generally show patients and the
family or friends representative slides: the average result as well as
prominent scarring. Illustrations in publications about this technique are also helpful.

I state unambiguously that it is a rare patient who, after the most
successful treatment with the argon laser, can go completely without makeup; seldom does the skin become absolutely normal.

The fact that the argon laser is new and represents an advance
does not necessarily mean that the patient will be ecstatic over even
a good result. Human expectations escalate and what may have
pleased the patient three months ago may no longer suffice. The
patient wants not only more but better.

In evaluating these patients psychologically, Kalick [82] observed,

Port wine stain patients seeking laser treatment generally have adapted
reasonably well to their medical condition. Those past adolescence are
likely to have married and/or made progress in their career. Still, they feel
plagued by the "birth mark" they feel they have unfairly had to bear.
Many patients look upon the laser as a magic ray which will redeem them
of their burden. They must be bluntly informed of the chance of scarring,
the likely incomplete fading, and the short term injury done by the laser.
These are aspects of treatment the chance of which they would prefer not
to discover and, if given the opportunity, it will readily ignore.

FINANCES

Many insurance plans now cover argon laser treatment, especially
in children. Except for those very young, the argon laser exposure
can be accomplished on an outpatient basis with the use of local
anesthesia. Some centers now have the facilities for laser treatment
in the operating room, where children can receive general anesthesia.

AFTER TREATMENT

The patient and the family receive printed instructions (see Appendix) concerning the management of the skin area after laser therapy. Pain is usually very minimal or absent and the care of the wound is relatively simple. Assessing the final result from laser treatment requires six months to a year. Late improvement, even after a year, has been observed.

As mentioned, even when the test patch portends a favorable result, there is no guarantee that further treatment will produce the same result or will not produce scarring. The decision as to whether to proceed must ultimately be made by the patient in conjunction with family and friends and you. Since I have close family members or friends in the room at the time the patient is receiving the laser treatment, there is already a togetherness for this project.

As with every congenital abnormality, the patient may fear that he or she will be its progenitor. Only in comparatively rare instances does the port wine stain represent an inheritable trait. An open discussion about the genetics of this condition may relieve the patient, especially if of marriageable age, of an enormous anxiety.

Skin Lesions

For those doing general plastic and reconstructive surgery, cutaneous lesions constitute a large proportion of their work. They are the bread and butter of a practice, especially for a beginner. To the surgeon, most of these skin growths are minimal problems but to the patient and/or the referring doctor, they are major considerations; otherwise that person would not be in a plastic surgeon's office.

For the young doctor who has just completed his or her residency, the facial lesion may be the test case, whether or not he or she knows it. The referring doctor and the patient will judge the young surgeon's performance in this minor situation before entrusting him or her with something of greater magnitude, such as a breast reconstruction or a facelift. They will evaluate him or her not only by the final scar but by his or her personality as a physician. Treating these modest lesions thus is a means of becoming known in the community. In the same amount of time as required for an augmentation mammoplasty, for example (which involves only one patient), you can remove growths from five patients. Furthermore, patients who have facial lesions excised will discuss you and the operation with less reticence than they would if they had had a breast augmentation or a facelift. This form of advertising is appropriate and represents the safest base on which your practice should rest—patient referral.

In many instances, your removing a cutaneous lesion may save someone's life: for example, malignant melanoma or invasive squamous cell carcinoma. Remember that when you tell a patient that he or she has a skin "cancer" the patient will be understandably frightened. Just because an epithelioma might be routine to you, do not expect a patient to be equally placid about it. Far from it. Many patients can remember a relative or friend who died of "cancer"—in some instances, of a skin cancer. Take care to explain, if the circumstances warrant it, that a skin cancer such as a basal cell carcinoma does not have the same lethal potential as a cancer of the lung, breast, or stomach. In some instances, it is wise to telephone the patient's spouse or parent to give reassurance on that point. With regard to a small, untreated basal cell carcinoma, you should emphasize that the probability of cure is about 98 percent and that the patient will not likely be severely disfigured or scarred from the disease or your treatment. Obviously, these statements can be made only if they are objectively justified. With a malignant melanoma, of course, the situation is different and undiluted optimism would be misleading.

In general, the surgical care of these lesions is excision under local anesthesia, on an outpatient basis either at your office or at the hospital. Usually the patient's insurance will pay for the procedure. If the patient is a subscriber to a group Blue Cross/Blue Shield plan, in many states you are not allowed to bill beyond what you are paid. Though these rules may seem unfair, especially if the recompense has been small, they must be honored.

BIOPSY

Until recently, I did an excisional biopsy if I suspected a basal cell carcinoma unless the lesion was located in a difficult area of the face, such as the eyelid or nasal tip. However, because of legal considerations, I now obtain an incisional biopsy of large lesions so I can explain alternatives of treatment to the patient, who then knows the precise diagnosis. Some patients emotionally can never tolerate a scar, no matter how fine it is. For them, radiation therapy may be a good alternative. I arrange a consultation with a respected therapist so the patient will get information about the advantages and disadvantages of the method as well as about the number of sessions necessary over what length of time, about the possibility of recurrence, and about radiation changes in the tissues, from loss of pigmentation to necrosis.

Patients must be warned that occasionally a wide excision of an area diagnosed by biopsy to be a basal cell carcinoma will now show malignancy. Unless the patient understands about the "disappearance" of the epithelioma, you will be accused of unnecessary surgery [65].

For every benign lesion, the surgeon and the patient should ask themselves why excision is being considered. Frequently, no operation should be done as, for example, for a harmless-looking nevus or growth on the sternum or cheek. Beware of the patient who wants it removed for "cosmetic reasons." Although this is understandable as a motivation, the patient might be disappointed by the resulting scar. It is interesting and sometimes surprising that the person who has lived with an ugly lesion may have great difficulty in adjusting to a scar—even a good one. One must be certain to tell the patient there is no guaranteeing what type of scar he or she will have and that it will take several months to determine whether the scar is favorable or unfavorable. One must be wary also of operating on parts of the body that have an inclination to form hypertrophic scars or keloids: the sternum, the tip of the shoulder, or the neck—particularly in an adolescent. One also sometimes has to make the difficult decision as to how many nevi to remove; since most Caucasians have 10 to 30 "moles" on their body, it would be foolish to attempt excising them all. Occasionally, to allay your anxiety and that of the patient and the family about not doing enough, a consultation with a dermatologist is helpful.

Be careful also of the patient who is having a lesion removed to please someone else. I remember a 25-year-old woman who wanted me to excise a small nevus of her chin. It was so inconspicuous that I asked her why she wanted this done now. The reason, she said, was that she was to be married in two months and her fiancé, a photographer, "couldn't stand the looks of it." In probing, I elicited other instances of his making her feel insecure about herself. Tearfully, she admitted her concerns about this aspect of their relationship. Of course, I refused to operate but did suggest that she rethink her decision about matrimony.

PREOPERATIVE CONSIDERATIONS

UNDERESTIMATING THE PROBLEM. The Russian proverb is apt. "More drown in puddles than in the sea." Removal of a skin lesion may seem simple surgically but occasionally closing the defect may cause you consternation and embarrassment. A flap or graft may be required, a possibility that you had not contemplated when you initially saw the patient; you may not have properly informed him or her then of this eventuality. Therefore, think carefully about any patient with a lesion and avoid the unpleasant situation of being unprepared in the operating room.

Another error is to subject patients to excision on an outpatient basis under local anesthesia when, in reality, they should have been admitted and operated on either with local anesthesia and intravenous supplementation or with general anesthesia. For the patient who is elderly or anxious, outpatient surgery may not be advisable. In taking the history, inquire about the patient's reaction to previous local anesthesia. Often, patients will tell you frankly that they cannot stand needles and faint whenever they go to the dentist. Sometimes these patients can endure local anesthesia on an outpatient basis but frequently they cannot. You must ask also about previous cardiovascular disease, palpitations, and current medications. It may be necessary for you to consult the patient's cardiologist or internist before deciding that the operation can be done on an outpatient basis with local anesthesia containing epinephrine, even in reduced amounts. Some older patients with facial lesions look healthy, but you may find out that they have not had a thorough physical examination in many years. You then must either refer them to an internist or family doctor or examine them yourself and then order a complete blood count, urinalysis, chest x ray, and electrocardiogram.

Almost every patient with a facial lesion worries about the scar and may think that you, the plastic surgeon, can do scarless surgery. The reality will be an unpleasant shock. With the patient looking into the mirror, demonstrate the excision you plan by outlining it with a skin marker. If the lesion is a basal cell carcinoma, you can explain to the patient why it is necessary to remove a larger area than the apparent growth. You also can outline a flap that you might be using. Indicate also where the scars will be and reiterate that they will be permanent.

Many patients believe that plastic surgeons either use plastic or a skin graft so there will be no scarring. Disabuse them of these misconceptions by pointing out that a skin graft will always look like a patch, most likely depressed and of different color than the surrounding skin; and that ideally the best closure is bringing the edges of the skin together if there is sufficient tissue. If necessary, a flap may be chosen to supply skin and you can discuss its advantages: a better match in color, contour, and texture than a skin graft.

A skin graft, however, may be indicated. Inform the patient as to the location of the donor site, how it will heal, and what type of scar it will leave. Be certain the patient understands that there is a chance the graft will fail and another procedure may be necessary a couple of weeks later. Because grafting is a common procedure for us, do not forget that it is unusual for patients. They have probably read about it and consider it mysterious and magical.

INSTRUCTIONS TO THE PATIENT.   I tell these and all preoperative patients in words and in writing not to take aspirin or aspirin-containing compounds for 10 days before operation so that they will have normal clotting.

Patients are also instructed not to eat or drink for eight hours before their procedure if it is to last more than a half-hour. The anesthesia departments in most hospitals have rules for outpatient surgery. While many of their stipulations may seem unnecessary and excessive, the patient will be safer medically and you, legally, if these rules have been followed.

DURING OPERATION

Wherever the procedure is done, lighting and facilities must be optimal. Doing a small operation under unfavorable circumstances may convert it into an unpleasant big operation. The patient should have vital signs taken initially and periodically; older patients should have cardiac monitoring and an electrocardiograph running continuously. These precautions may seem superfluous but it is better to prevent a problem than suddenly to have to remedy it and occasionally to be unable even to do that.

Your operation will be better for all concerned if the patient is relaxed. Avoid any discussion that might cause worry, blood pressure rise, and bleeding increase. Since the patient is awake, he or she is aware of all stimuli. Try to minimize unnecessary noise and the parade of personnel in and out of the operating room.

As the surgeon, you are ultimately responsible for the lesion reaching the pathologist. If more than one has been removed, each should be labeled separately. Complete the pathologist's forms yourself or have a responsible person do it but never assign this task to someone unfamiliar with the patient's history or with medical terminology.

AFTER OPERATION

Instructions to the patient should be clear and, preferably, written so the patient and/or family and friends can be certain of what you want and what they should do. The patient should be told about the pain to expect and should be given something to counteract it. Again inquire about sensitivities to medicines.

The patient should know about the care of the dressing: in general, not to wet it. If you wish it changed, give the patient those instructions along with supplies. If the operation was performed in the area around the mouth, you may not wish to allow the patient to chew for a day or two. It would have been wise to inform the patient of this possibility prior to the operation so that he or she could have made proper arrangements at home and also could have refused social invitations where those restrictions might prove embarrassing. Either make an appointment with the patient to remove the sutures, or have him or her call your office to obtain one.

How the patient goes home is an important consideration. At the time of the initial consultation, you should have discussed this aspect and instructed patients to have someone drive them home if you felt that they should not do it themselves. No matter how slight the operation, every patient has anxiety about it. In addition, the local anesthesia may have changed the patient's normal body responses. If, at the conclusion of the procedure, the patient is not perfectly fit to leave the hospital or your office, keep that patient until there is no question about his or her safety in returning home. You should also know who will be at home to care for the patient. Sometimes it is essential that the patient be closely observed, particularly if very young or old or if there is a history of a systemic problem such as hypertension, epilepsy, or diabetes. If you have concerns about the patient's being able to go home, do not allow it, even if you had not discussed this possibility when you initially saw him or her at your office. Do not make two errors. Admit that you had not paid sufficient heed to the patient's physical condition or the availability of supervision at home. About once every couple of years, a patient unexpectedly must remain overnight in the hospital. Although this decision may cause consternation for the patient and his family, it is preferable to later mourning another lapse in judgment.

Reduction of Nasal Fracture

The reader might be surprised by my including in this book the seemingly simple procedure of reducing a fractured nose. Perhaps because of its presumed simplicity, the patient may erroneously expect a perfect result unless properly forewarned by the surgeon. My contention is that this operation has more unfavorable results than are generally appreciated.

Several factors are responsible: The surgeon called in to treat the patient with a nasal fracture never knows precisely what the patient's nose really looked like before the accident. The patient usually claims that it was perfectly straight. Sometimes looking at the patient's photo on a driver's license or an identification card can give one some idea of the preexisting shape of the nose.

Frequently the surgeon schedules reduction of the nasal fracture at a time convenient for him or her but not optimal for obtaining the best result. Many patients arrive in the emergency room at night and they are scheduled for reduction 24 to 48 hours later, when the swelling is at its maximum and is obscuring the anatomical landmarks.

Often the nasal fracture is reduced under inadequate conditions of poor lighting and meager facilities (absence of suction and proper instruments). One patient told me that she had gone to a plastic surgeon who "seemed annoyed that he had to fit me into his office schedule. He did it right there in his office but he didn't wait for the Novocain to work. The pain was awful and my nose is as crooked as it was before he tried to fix it."

That patient's tale does emphasize the fact that the least a patient should expect from a doctor is a caring attitude about the pain involved with any procedure.

Every patient must be told that after reduction, the nose may not be what it was prior to the trauma and that another operation, perhaps six months later, may be necessary to straighten it. I inform each patient and the family that I shall try to put back what goes back easily but I never use "brute force" to align the nose for fear of distorting it or causing hemorrhage or both. Occasionally, even when the nose has been properly reduced, bleeding can persist and may require packing and, in rare instances, ligation of the external carotid or anterior ethmoidal artery.

Always inquire about the patient's past history with regard to hypertension and medications such as aspirin and anticoagulants.

Using local and topical anesthesia is customary but some patients, particularly adolescents, are quite anxious about the operation although they pretend otherwise. Intravenous supplementation is helpful but it should not be given unless the patient has been without food or drink for at least six to eight hours. Of course, with smaller children, it may be necessary to administer general anesthesia, whose risks should also be explained to the parents.

Other Facial Fractures

I shall not go into detail concerning the interaction between the plastic surgeon and the patient with fractures of the face in addition to that of the nose. What I wish to stress here is the need for awareness of any associated injuries (see p. 185) as well as disruption of other facial bones, besides the obvious fracture. Furthermore, the treatment of facial trauma may require the convergence of talent: oral surgeon, ophthalmologist, otolaryngologist, and neurosurgeon, in addition to plastic surgeon. The patient should never be the victim of the unfortunate internecine battles among specialties.

Another point for emphasis is to tell the patient, if alert and comprehending, as well as the family, what your operative approach will be and its expected success. For example, in the instance of a zygomatic fracture, the patient should know whether you are planning a Gillies or transantral reduction or an incision into the cheek with direct wiring, if indicated. In the press of an emergency, it is easy to forget or not to take the time to give adequate information. Rushing the patient into the operating room is seldom warranted and can cause catastrophe if, for example, there is unsuspected systemic illness or unrecognized damage to the eye or brain.

It is wise to state your disclaimers before the operation. You probably should warn the patient and the family that he or she may never have the same bony configuration or soft-tissue covering as existed before the accident. Furthermore, additional operations may be necessary. Once the patient has recovered from the emotional shock of having sustained facial trauma, the gratitude that you think he or she will exhibit may disappear in the patient's disappointment that things are not perfect. The unhappy patient might reason that "if plastic surgeons can put back arms and legs, why couldn't they get my face to looking like it was before?" If you are able to remind the patient and the family about the fact that you mentioned the limitations of the operation before you performed it, energies will not go into defending yourself but into helping the patient readapt.

Head and Neck Surgery

Most plastic surgeons in the United States are seeing decreased numbers of patients with tumors of the head and neck. The reasons are multiple: decreased incidence of the disease; different methods are managing malignancy, such as irradiation instead of surgery; fewer plastic surgeons who are able and wish to care for these patients; and the availability of other specialists to perform the surgery (otolaryngologists and general surgeons).

Patients with head and neck neoplasms may have either benign or malignant disease. Aside from those with parotid tumors, patients with head and neck malignancy usually are men who disproportionately come from the lower socioeconomic groups and frequently have a history of poor oral hygiene, excessive smoking, and alcohol intake.

In general, these patients are seen more often in hospital clinics than in private offices in contrast to those for cosmetic surgery. Patients with parotid tumors, however, usually go to private surgeons.

No one with intraoral malignancy can be treated so easily or reassured so fully as someone with a basal cell carcinoma of the skin. With the former, the morbidity, mortality, and deformity are significant. Even with the newest techniques of reconstruction, utilizing musculocutaneous flaps and microsurgical transfer of tissue, the patient's appearance is forever altered, always for the worse. Furthermore, speech and swallowing may be impaired.

In a private office, the patient is usually accompanied by a member of the family. At the clinic, he or she may be alone; this should make the surgeon realize that the patient will have to depend more upon him or her for support since the emotional cushion of family or friends may not be available.

In taking the history and systems review, you must remember that the condition of the patient is potentially, if not actually, serious and the treatment will be major. An operation such as a resection of the floor of the mouth and a portion of the mandible, with a radical neck dissection, significantly stresses that patient's soma as well as psyche. Since those with head and neck malignancy are in the older age groups, their general health will be the principal factor in the selection of their treatment and its success or failure. In addition, as mentioned, these patients tend to drink and to smoke excessively. Since their cardiopulmonary status may not be optimal, they must be properly evaluated for anesthesia and surgery. Inquire also about fatigue, weight loss, appetite, and social habits, including their work. As you are asking these questions, try to ascertain what impact the disease and treatment will have on all aspects of the patient's life.

PHYSICAL EXAMINATION

No matter what or where the primary lesion, your physical examination must be thorough with regard to the entire head and neck: presence or absence of palpable nodes, status of the facial nerve, and condition of the teeth. Indirect laryngoscopy is mandatory for evaluation of the mouth, pharynx, and vocal cords. Is there any other primary lesion? Since extensive surgery is being contemplated, these patients must have their blood pressure taken as well as their heart, lungs, and abdomen examined.

INFORMING THE PATIENT

If you think the patient will require surgery that you rarely do or are uncomfortable in performing, now is the time to refer (see p. 53).

You must inform the patient of your tentative diagnosis. Perhaps the diagnosis is known; maybe a biopsy is needed. If you believe that the patient will definitely require an operation, discuss it in detail but do not suddenly overwhelm him with a statement such as, "This means that I shall have to remove half your face and jaw." The same information can be given gradually and gently. Place yourself in that patient's position of fighting for survival while trying to preserve his features as a human being. Sometimes it is better to defer telling the hard facts if you sense that the patient cannot take it all at once or if he is alone in your office; a better occasion may be when a spouse or sibling, for example, can be there. Offer to see the patient in a day or two when his usual source of support can be present.

If you believe the best treatment of the lesion is irradiation and surgery or irradiation alone, arrange for the patient to see the radiotherapist. Perhaps the patient should be evaluated by the oncology group at your hospital. These are not useless maneuvers. The patient and you usually will gain from other opinions and a discussion of possible alternatives. He will then be able to accept your recommendations, feeling that you have not neglected anything or anyone in attempting to help. It also will give you more assurance for the course you are taking.

Allow time for the patient to ask some questions. Basic to his inquiries is a pervasive concern that the resulting deformity will be so great that even if he is well, he will no longer be welcomed in society and will be an embarrassment to family and friends. Sometimes the surgeon can call upon patients who went through similar procedures and have offered to see other patients facing their type of surgery. Laryngectomy groups, for example, are extremely helpful. Hearing it from others who have been there before can be a tremendous source of confidence for the patient and his or her family. Remember that the face is sacrosanct: It is basic to the self-image of each of us. In every other situation in life, we instinctively try to protect our face. In this instance, the patient must sacrifice a part of it in order to live. The fact that you have done 50 commando procedures does not lessen the impact for the patient, for whom this is the first head and neck operation.

Almost every patient with a serious cancer, not a basal cell, however, feels a stigma. For most people, healthy or with malignancy, cancer means death, excruciating pain, something stealthy and dirty. This "metaphorical thinking," as Sontag [136] calls it, tends to isolate the person not only because of the reactions of others but also his or her own; the afflicted one withdraws through guilt, shame, and fear as if to spare his or her social circle of the task of dealing with a deviant. The doctor, of course, must do everything possible to prevent the patient from becoming a pariah. If, indeed, a patient who has had a hidden cancer treated (e.g., cancer of the colon removed by colectomy) experiences depression and a desire to run away, one can get some idea of what the patient with a head and neck cancer must endure. That individual has to bear the visible signs of the exorcisation of this dread disease. Despite the tremendous stress that a head and neck malignancy imposes on an individual, the incidence of suicide is very low, less than 0.05 percent [27]—a tribute to the courage and adaptability of the human being.

BEFORE OPERATION

Be meticulous about your preparation of patients for surgery. Warn them not to take aspirin or aspirin-containing compounds. Perhaps they will need a high-protein diet in preparation for the ordeal. They may require also determination of blood gases and chest physical therapy because of many years of cigarette smoking and the presence of emphysema and bronchitis. A consultation with the anesthesiologist before the patient is admitted to the hospital may prevent a frustrating night-before cancellation because of insufficient workup.

IN THE HOSPITAL

Although there are many things that could be discussed here depending upon the procedure, the major consideration is your responsibility to help patients accept themselves and their new appearance, as well as perhaps altered speech and swallowing. Be there at the first dressing change. Do not abandon them at this critical time. Help them to look in the mirror and support them through the shock of seeing somebody new in the mirror, somebody who looks ugly and foreign to them. Most patients' immediate concern is appearance, not function—not survival, even though you may think it should be otherwise. Be careful of the patient who says, "My appearance doesn't really bother me." Perhaps that is true but more likely he is trying to hide deep concern from you. Such a response may be a result of guilt about expressing displeasure with his appearance when you have tried so hard to save his life.

The presence of sympathetic nurses is important to any patient. For a man, the female nurse or female doctor will be the first woman to see his new face without dressings. If they do not grimace or turn away but relate calmly to him, this will considerably strengthen his self-esteem. In World War II, McIndoe knew well the value of this kind of social reintegration when he provided female companionship for his facially burned RAF pilots [151].

The patient who has had extensive remodeling of the intestine—as, for example, after a Whipple procedure—cannot see what the surgeon has done because of the fortunate covering of the abdominal wall. The patient who has had serious head and neck surgery eventually must go unveiled.

FOLLOW-UP
Your responsibility to the patient continues for his or her lifetime. The issue is not just survival at 5, 10, or 15 years, but resumption of normal living and relationships. A clue to how things are going at home is whether there has been a change in sexual relations with the spouse. Have they been able to get together? If not, why not? Sometimes the partner is willing but the patient feels worthless. Your intervention or that of a skilled family therapist may make a considerable difference in the lives of the entire family. In many ways, it is easier for a physician when the cancer is the only enemy. After surgery, the battle must be waged against more elusive opponents, sometimes harder to defeat. With more reconstruction, the patient's appearance can be improved but ultimately there is a limit. At that point, the patient hopefully has been able to adapt. If not, referral to a psychiatrist and/or support groups of similar patients might rescue him or her from the downward spiral of depression.

Another point to mention is the necessity of an adequate postoperative follow-up. Too often, these examinations are perfunctory. Unconsciously, the surgeon does not wish to find recurrent or new disease. However, there is no point in examining that patient unless the surgeon is willing to find what is there and to act upon it. Periodic evaluations by the local tumor group or the oncology group may be a helpful supplement to your care of the patient. However, the primary responsibility for your patient's management should not be shifted to someone else unless there is just cause. You have become, and should remain, that patient's doctor.

The Pediatric Patient
This heading was carefully chosen since the stages of infancy, childhood, youth, and maturity are arbitrary and indistinct, not

only chronologically but physically and emotionally as well. Presently most of my patients are adults but I once had a brisk pediatric practice.

The pediatric patient is not an adult in miniature any more than an elderly patient is an aged child. A child has characteristics common to all children but also traits that are unique.

From a practical viewpoint, what is special about treating pediatric patients?

1. They do not usually come of their own volition. Parents or surrogates bring them.

2. In general, the earlier a deformity is corrected, the better the psychological effects (perhaps also the anatomical results) in a child. This axiom relates to the important aspects of body image and self-esteem. Quality of life for someone with Apert's syndrome, for example, would be significantly enhanced if the disfiguring abnormalities were improved before 2 years of age rather than at the age of 14. Of course, this surgical objective is not always attainable. We should remember also that the importance to psychic development of being different is not restricted only to facial features; any part, especially if abnormal, may be emotionally important to a particular person: webbed fingers, asymmetric breasts, a conspicuous nevus or hemangioma of the trunk.

3. Very young children cannot verbally communicate their symptoms or concerns. Even when children can talk, their speech is not so elaborate as that of adults; however, in a few stark phrases, they may convey more that is meaningful and true than a 44-year-old, who has learned to dissimulate feelings and to bury anxiety and hostility under a cloak of words. Compared to an adult, the child rationalizes less. Whereas children are affected by what they may have seen on television or read in books, adults more frequently describe themselves and their sentiments in terms of what they think they should be or feel.

To go to the core of a child is easier than to reach that of an adult, who has a much thicker carapace. For many adults, one is tempted to ask, "Will the real Mrs. _____ stand up?" But not so with a pediatric patient. That is not to say that children cannot be devious in action and speech. They can, but more commonly the surgeon who is used to adults may be caught off guard by a child's direct expression of feeling—such as tantrums, crying spells, sudden physical and emotional withdrawal.

A child, however, may be a better reader of body language than an adult. Perhaps this comes from a child's having to look so often at big people and having to judge quickly, for self-preservation, what that person may do either to harm or to help him. We might get a sense of that vulnerability by imagining ourselves in the company of the entire Pittsburgh Steelers team.

The more "intellectual" the adult (and being intellectual usually takes years), the more labyrinthian his or her thought. Adults may pride themselves on their subtlety and on their ability to emit double-entendres, to be clever with a forked tongue. Generally not so with a child, who is always on the important side of the decimal point.

Think straight, talk straight, and act straight should be our maxim with all patients, but especially with children. One can be direct without being abrupt or uncaring. Telling a child that a needle stick will not hurt and is "like a mosquito bite" (rather than a bee sting) is a foolish lie. This breach of the truth may make the child distrust everything you subsequently say or do. Far better to inform the child that there will be pain but that it is momentary but necessary for you to help with the problem.

4. Just as adults do better in a hospital with other adults, children fare better with other children in a pediatric hospital or ward. The staff are more familiar with their needs. Children feel secure knowing that they are in an environment dedicated to them. Not all doctors or nurses or all adults enjoy being with children and children sense their irritation and hostility. Another advantage of a pediatric unit is the decreased likelihood of errors in medication from personnel more accustomed to managing adult patients.

5. When contemplating surgery in children, one must think in terms of future growth and development; whereas in adults, the consideration is aging.

For the child with a cleft lip and palate, the surgeon must question whether the procedure will interfere with normal maturation. When performing a facelift, the surgeon hopes that the procedure will interfere with the normal sequence of aging.

The variables of growth and development can surprise the surgeon: A result that looks good in an infant may look bad when the person is a teenager. Occasionally, the opposite occurs, particularly with scars.

6. Follow-up examination may mean something different to a child than to an adult.

A child, for example, who has had a cleft lip repaired at 3 months of age may not wish to see his surgeon every year because he fears another operation. The parents, in some instances, may not even have told the child that he had a cleft lip but attributed the scar to a fall when he was a baby. The child who knows about the cleft lip may become self-conscious with an excessive number of follow-up visits, especially if his or her result is good and awareness of the problem is minimal.

An older patient, however, after a breast reduction or augmentation or after an eyelidplasty or facelift may welcome return visits because they are reassuring and also offer the occasion to ask for more surgery. In fact, as was mentioned earlier, for this reason, some surgeons do not wish to follow their patients for a long time; they want to avoid expressions of dissatisfaction and pleas for touch-up operations.

7. Pediatric patients, in general, are less capable of following directions or performing their own dressing changes than adults.

A child of 4, as an example, cannot be expected to remember to take medication or to change dressings alone. Most children are fortunate to have parental reminding and assistance. Also, children who are normally active may make a shambles of a dressing or a cast; that situation in an adult occurs less often.

8. Because the relationship between children and parents is generally close, it is rare for a child to pursue an operation without parental support. This is certainly not the situation with older patients, who may seek surgery against the advice and wishes of their family. The teenager, however, is in a revolutionary phase of life and may act in much the same way as the older, so-called liberated woman. The problem is that the older patient has society's support as well as its legal sanction to proceed with treatment, but not so a child or a young teenager.

Although it is unwise in most surgical situations with adults not to have an operation become a family affair, it is almost impossible to avoid this when a child is concerned. That is why the surgeon with pediatric patients must be very much attuned to family dynamics.

Many hospitals have programs to make surgery less anxiety-provoking for children: preadmission tours, even parties, and films allow parents, siblings, prospective patients, and their friends to become familiar with what will happen during their hospitalization. Pediatric patients, like many adults, have a particular fear of anesthesia and the opportunity to talk to an anesthetist, to see and examine the equipment, markedly reduces their anxiety. Having facilities to accommodate a parent is also a major plus or should be for the child and for you. Occasionally a parent, by his or her presence, may increase the child's fears. Frequently also the nursing staff may resent what they consider to be the intrusion of the parent in their province. Of course, it is the parent's child, not theirs, but this type of proprietary thinking on the part of a nurse is not all bad: It may be responsible for laudatory dedication to the welfare of those in his or her care.

A common mistake of many physicians is to attempt to reassure a child by hugging and kissing when you don't know each other. The child will instinctively retreat from this inappropriate and overwhelming advance. Proceed slowly but gently. In any relationship, it takes time to build trust.

The Paraplegic Patient

The purpose of this section is not to describe the many procedures used for resurfacing a decubitus ulcer. Rather, it is to share some thoughts concerning the management of paraplegic patients.

The most common error made by plastic surgeons treating a paraplegic patient is to place too much faith in a flap and to pay insufficient attention to the psyche. Commonly, we consult on an individual who has had numerous episodes of sacral breakdown and many previous reconstructive procedures. At this time, the use of musculocutaneous flaps is popular but we must resist the temptation in our residents and ourselves to do this operation without understanding the etiology of the ulcer. I am not referring to the question of pressure or shearing force but something more fundamental. Has the patient been self-destructive? Do the repeated incidents of breakdown reflect a depression, an escape into alcoholism, a desire to re-enter the hospital because the outside world is too much to confront? Having been a consultant on a spinal cord injury service, I was impressed that some patients, fortunately only a small percentage, returned repeatedly to the hospital after having left healed; in every instance, the fault was not with the flap but in the mind of the patient. It is fruitless to expect that a new flap will provide indefinite protection when the patient refuses to cooperate in his or her own care. This type of patient needs counseling or group support and, frequently, prolonged psychotherapy. If the patient had seen a psychiatrist early in the course of his or her overwhelming disability, then some of these later psychological problems might either not have arisen or might have been less severe.

Often when we are called by another physician to see these patients, they are lying on their abdomen and seldom do we go to the head of the bed to look at their faces and to talk with them before snatching off their dressing and outlining a flap. We treat them as an ulcer, not as a human being. Our attitude reinforces their low self-esteem and their hostility toward themselves and the world. It would be naive to assume that a plastic surgeon—even the most compassionate, understanding, and skilled—could reverse a damaging psychological sequence. However, at least he or she need not add to it. The plastic surgeon who comprehends the patient as a human being will avoid surgery that is doomed to failure. During the time that an ulcer is cleaning up or healing in, an effort should be made to view and treat these patients globally so that subsequent surgery will not be a mere technical exercise for which the duration of success will be just a few months.

The Patient with Factitious Disease

The crux in the management of this difficult type of patient is to recognize the diagnosis. So accustomed are we to relieving patients of an unwanted disease that we may easily overlook the possibility that someone may wish to have an illness [114]. The patient, of course, has a psychological sickness in addition to the one that is simulated.

Psychological classification of such patients, termed by some to have Münchausen's syndrome [102], is difficult and controversial. In my experience, patients have usually been women, 20 to 50 years of age, with a disproportionately large number in the medical field—nurses and technicians. A plastic surgeon will usually encounter such a patient because of failure of the wound to heal or recurrence of a local cutaneous infection. Since many patients are one of us—medical—we are reluctant to consider the factitious nature of the problem. They may be attractive, intelligent, and seemingly desirous to get well. Some may flatter you by saying that you are supposed to be "the best" and that is why they sought you. For some, their relationship to the physician becomes the center of their life and gratifies their prodigious dependency needs. This attachment may perpetuate their conscious or unconscious repeated simulation of physical disease. The physician is always uneasy in confronting a patient with evidence that he or she has manufactured illness. Yet at some point it may be necessary to do so, but only after psychiatric consultation and approval. These patients are notoriously refractory to treatment and some may die in the course of causing their disease. Suicide by another means is also a possibility. Curing a recurrent wound breakdown, for example, may not solve the major underlying problems since another focus may be chosen, one that may be even more dangerous to the patient's health.

A simple rule is to think of factitious disease whenever a patient repeatedly fails to respond to standard treatment for a relatively simple condition. Sometimes, you may have to intervene to treat the patient because of the disease that he or she has caused. Try to keep your interventions simple. Do a graft rather than a flap, if possible. Do not delude yourself with your own competence and your faith in the knife. Remember that the principal problem is cerebral and even if you are fortunate to "cure" the ostensible illness, your success may be short-lived. For the surgeon, these patients present the modern equivalent of a Hobson's choice.

When Things Have Gone Wrong

There are days and there are other days.
ANDRÉ GIDE
Autumn Leaves

THE DISSATISFIED PATIENT

The dissatisfied patient is as much a reality of surgical practice as is the satisfied patient [43, 63]. Although in a minority, the unhappy patient generally has a greater emotional impact, albeit unpleasant on the surgeon. No picture of the surgical landscape would be complete without showing the one who should have gotten away.

As physicians, we seek to help others and to obtain their approbation. It is distressing to have to deal with a person whom we not only have not helped but possibly have made worse; who, instead of being grateful, is hostile; and who, instead of applauding our motives and talents, openly accuses us of greed and incompetence.

A plastic surgical residency, like most other educational experiences in our culture, does not usually equip us to manage the unpleasant side of our metier. As residents, we took care of the grief of our attending surgeons and their patients, the rotation would soon be over or, like a deus ex machina, we might even be leaving town in a few months. But now, as professionals, we are all in a position so well described by Harry Truman. "The buck stops here."

The first task for the surgeon is to know when and why a patient is dissatisfied. Usually he or she will remove all ambiguity by a strong, unequivocal statement of complaint but if this is not forthcoming, we should be alert to veiled discontent—a sullenness, an irritability, or some form of passive-aggressive behavior such as not keeping appointments or not paying the bill if, unwisely, we asked no prepayment for an esthetic operation. In some ways, it seems easier to let the patient leave the office and we feel relief because he or she did not verbalize the unpleasantness we would then have to confront. But sooner or later the seamy side of surgery will have to be faced. We must not become so unreceptive that the patient's resentment will reach the proportions of a lethal abscess. Before this occurs a helpful comment might be, "You don't seem too happy today. What is troubling you?" Then step back as Pandora's box opens!

In truth, some patients seem more unhappy than they are. Unless they have told you what bothers them, sometimes asking them if there is anything that they like about the result may elicit a more positive response than you had thought possible. This becomes a good foundation upon which to build the ensuing discussion.

For many patients dissatisfaction disappears with reassurance that is justified by circumstances. For example, someone who is concerned two weeks after eyelidplasty about swelling can be told it will subside as healing progresses over the next few months. He or she may have to be reminded of that rare virtue, *patience*. A patient may worry about the bulkiness of a recently turned flap. Here, too, reassurance about progressive flattening will be comforting.

Occasionally, postoperative unhappiness centers on the minimal or the nonexistent. In this situation, it is important to probe into "why this now?" Is the person depressed and guilty about having an elective operation or about something else? Has there been a recent loss such as a divorce or death? I remember a 35-year-old married woman who had a very good result following a rhinoplasty and chin implant but seemed depressed a few weeks later. Her girlfriend next door, she told me, had "kept away" and finally confessed to my patient that she feared rejection because she thought that my patient, now better looking, would need her less. Occasionally the culprit in postoperative depression is the family physician, who may have said to the patient soon after a facelift, "you went through all this to look like that?" This unkind and destructive remark may have been prompted by the patient's not consulting him or her about the surgery or proceeding without advice. In addition, the general practitioner or internist may feel that the surgical fee is excessive compared to what he or she receives for the care of that same individual. Envy and jealousy, although not usually openly discussed, are relevant when managing a dissatisfied patient.

In this regard another factor to consider is the spouse or lover who may have enjoyed the personal dominance that resulted partly from the mate's feelings of inferiority about a disliked feature. Since she or he is now rid of it, the partner may feel less secure about the leverage he or she formerly possessed.

What about the patient who complains legitimately about an undesirable result; for example, infection, asymmetry, or bad scarring? To detail the spectrum of complications is beyond the present task and unnecessary for the purpose here. The point is that if the patient's dissatisfaction has an objective basis it, like any reality, deserves the surgeon's attention and respect and the patient merits our sympathy. Someone who has had esthetic surgery, for example, frequently has sought it against the advice of family, friends, and other physicians and may have had to pay for it personally. When something goes wrong, he or she feels foolish, ashamed, guilty, and angry. The patient may believe that this complication is divine recompense for vanity that led to risking health for a "frivolous improvement" that now has become a distinct liability.

As surgeons, especially since most of our results are favorable, we instinctively turn away from the adverse outcome but the sooner we accept it, the better we can manage it [19, 20]. To become angry at the patient because of our ego's bruise will succeed only in increasing hostility. The duet will soon become a duel. It is much better to recognize the reality and to work together to correct it. An unfavorable result happens not just to the patient but also to the family, to the surgeon, and, I might add, to the surgeon's family. Do not distort reality by accusing the patient of incorrect observation. The patient is certainly capable of judging nipple asymmetry, for example, or a bulbous tip or a "keloid" (which usually is a hypertrophic scar).

It is important that a plan of action be outlined as quickly as possible, and this may include what seemingly is no action. By that I mean that if one must wait before corrective surgery, that is still a plan and the patient will not feel forlorn or lost in ambiguity if it is so stated. Often I have told patients that the most difficult thing for us both is to wait. This requires restraint to avoid embarking precipitously on another operation that may compound the problem.

Not only should the patient be fully informed, but so should all pertinent members of the family and the referring physician or, if none, the family doctor. You and the patient need every ally possible.

When I first went into practice, a plastic surgeon told me that whenever something did not turn out right, he never admitted it to the patient and instructed everyone in his office to do the same. In this way, he thought, the patient would not consider him negligent and the hazard of a malpractice suit would be less. I cannot disagree more strongly with that precept. Although I would not advise beating our breasts, wearing ashes and sackcloth, and crying "mea culpa," I do not think that pretending the problem does not exist or lying to cover one's tracks will ever be justified from either a practical or moral standpoint. Several patients have told me that what infuriated them the most was seeing their physician as a dishonest human being. No one wants his doctor to be the Artful Dodger. Unfortunately, this kind of person exists not only in Dickens' novels. It was Mark Twain who wrote, "The truth is what you tell when you can't think of anything else to say." Without sounding like an evangelist, I would state that the truth is not the last resort but the first approach; it clears the air and allows you to resume the task for which you have trained half a lifetime: caring for a patient without being encumbered by shoddy stratagems that ultimately fail.

Another cardinal "don't" is to make yourself unavailable. Do not erect a barrier between you and the patient. The unfavorable result may actually be an opportunity to deepen the relationship and sometimes can be converted from a potentially miserable disaster into a satisfying experience. It is interesting that over the years several patients who have developed postoperative problems and were managed with a modicum of decency actually became enthusiastic supporters and subsequently referred other patients. Incidentally, giving the patient your home telephone number, for example, may make her or him more secure and may result in fewer telephone calls. The secretaries must be instructed that for this patient, the "hot line" is always open. If this is not done, the hard-to-reach doctor will soon be replaced by the easy-to-reach attorney. But, medicolegal considerations aside, it does not seem fair that you should make yourself scarce after you have contracted to do a job that might not have turned out as either you or the buyer wanted. We would certainly resent this attitude if a carpenter came to our home to perform a task and behaved in that fashion; surely we have more obligations to a patient whose face or life is at stake.

Another aspect in managing the dissatisfied patient is the proper utilization of a consultant. Most patients want to remain with the original physician, but it can comfort the patient as well as the surgeon to have another opinion, especially if the case warrants it. You should sense when the patient wishes a consultation, and you should not make the patient jump hurdles to obtain one. However, the patient should not feel tossed off but directed to the other physician. I usually dictate a letter in the patient's presence stating what the problem is and that I would like his or her advice, which can be discussed freely with the patient. Occasionally, you may sense that a patient does not feel that he or she should pay for "your mistake." I would hope that we would consent to see patients for colleagues at no charge to maintain the delicate balance between the unhappy individual and the hard-pressed physician. If you, as the referring physician, believe that the patient should not be charged for the consultation, you should so inform the surgeon and offer to pay for the consultation yourself. Most of us, I am sure, would not allow a colleague to do so, but there is precedence for this practice. If a patient chooses to continue his or her care under another doctor, either the consultant or someone else, do not make the patient feel guilty. In similar situations, I have made sure that I knew when the patient was going into the hospital and have even called the patient in the hospital or at home afterward. The patient then realizes that you are truly interested in his or her well-being, and the doctor who has cared for the patient will also welcome your support and not feel that he or she has lost a professional friend.

Many patients have told me that when they have suggested to the doctor a "second opinion," the response has been hostile. A recent patient who had mild ectropion after eyelidplasty recalled that the surgeon "said that he never wanted to see me back if I went to someone else." That doctor's attitude was puerile and irrational since the patient was a reasonable person, justifiably concerned about her eyes, which fortunately improved simply by waiting.

To illustrate some points in the management of the dissatisfied patient, let me give a few clinical examples. The patients are from my own practice. It is always easier to pontificate from the safe vantage point of someone else's patients, but what follows represents my own misadventures.

One problem situation involved a 58-year-old woman who, following a facelift, developed a moderate hematoma that was drained but left her with pathognomonic wrinkling. Over a few months this subsided, as did her feelings of hostility and anger, but it required twice weekly, then weekly visits and also a consultation with another plastic surgeon—which I initiated. I took periodic photographs to document the progress that she was making and I would show these to her. The patient, who had not prepaid her entire bill (my mistake), asked that a small amount remain unpaid because she said that she had not obtained the result she had expected and that she had endured considerable anxiety and stress in achieving what she got. Contrary to what the advice of some attorneys might be, I thought it reasonable to bend a little and our relations have been amicable since.

The second patient is the kind of woman about whom our residents ask, and very rightfully, "Why are you doing her?" She had a depressed air and, indeed, she was depressed to a degree that I did not appreciate; she had not recovered sufficiently from her son's death several years before. When she requested a facelift, she said she wanted to get out more, to feel better about herself, and, even though she was in her early 60s, she wanted to look for a job. This seemed reasonable but postoperatively she complained and still does, four years later, of vague discomfort, stiffness, and unusual sweating in her neck. She has seen a neurologist, a neurosurgeon, an orthopedic surgeon, a psychologist, and a psychiatrist—as well as another plastic surgeon. I have directed most of these referrals. She calls me from time to time and complains and then seems better after she has discussed it with me. The operation, with its unfortunate mysterious sequelae, has replaced her need to obtain employment. She represents an outstanding example of poor patient selection but also lingering distress of a patient, to whom the surgeon does have the obligation of "sticking with it." Fortunately, I have prevented her from seeking further surgery, which would prove even more deleterious to her well-being.

Mrs. W. is someone I remember well. She had an area of skin loss following a facelift. She was disappointed only to a minor degree, and with daily care the wound healed so that in that area behind the ear, the scarring was not very noticeable. She even sent a few of her friends to me after the operation. However, she returned a year or two later complaining that the scar hurt her severely. She seemed depressed and wondered how much the operation had really improved her appearance. Although the result may not have been outstanding, it certainly was more than acceptable. With this type of patient who is dissatisfied, it is necessary to probe, and indeed I found out that she had been very close to a married man who now was dying of cancer. She admitted that she wanted to speak to me again because she thought I might be sympathetic to her personal problems and probably this symptom of scar pain was really a pretext and a displacement. She wrote me later that her life was better; her friend had responded "remarkably well" to chemotherapy, and she no longer had pain behind the ear.

As physicians we know that pain is subjective, felt only by that individual who claims its presence. Since people vary widely in their pain tolerance, it is impossible to know precisely how much discomfort another person is truly having. Excessive pain after cosmetic surgery heralds a complication: hematoma, infection, or, if after eyelidplasty, perhaps impending blindness. Chronic pain after esthetic procedures is also infrequent. It may signify a depressed or displeased patient. The busy plastic surgeon, if not vigilant, may prescribe diazepam, for example, in a "get off my back" response to a patient's complaining and listlessness. Without probing for an explanation of that patient's mood, the surgeon may perpetuate and aggravate the despondency by giving a tranquilizer. With patients after reconstruction, a persistent pain, requiring analgesics and allegedly preventing return to work, should make you suspect malingering for secondary gain to collect on workmen's compensation or to garner a large settlement in court. Depression is also a possibility. Make an effort to determine the dynamics of that patient's behavior.

Always record what you prescribe and check before giving more for pain or sleep. Count your prescriptions. I remember two patients in whom I noted a disquieting fondness for sleeping pills. After I told them of my concern, they agreed to stop what they thought was "just a habit." Indeed, it was. The physician is also susceptible to a habit—that of prescribing without thinking.

Another clinical memory concerns someone on whom I did a facelift—someone who seemed to be a very cheerful human being but who I now realize was in a manic or hypomanic phase. She had had a daughter who had died in an auto accident two years before and had been seeing a psychiatrist who felt that she was handling her grief well and was out of the doldrums. About a year after the facelift, I was given an urgent message in the operating room to call her. She told me in no uncertain terms that she had the worst facelift of any of her friends. I remembered that she was given to bouts of excessive alcohol intake, although she sounded rational but obviously disturbed. I asked her to come to the office and later, after a long discussion, I did a revision of her eyelidplasty—right upper lid. A few months after this, she returned—again hostile and complaining—could I do anything further? I told her frankly that since she felt the surgery had not been what she wanted, it would be risky for us both to participate in another operating room adventure. It is difficult to break off with a patient, but I think sometimes it is necessary or the downtrend will continue as a *folie à deux*.

Every so often we see a patient who has had surgery, such as a facelift, and at the time of follow-up visit we forget that we have already done her. She looks as if she is in the office for a facelift and it is embarrassing to realize that the improvement you both had expected never materialized. Sometimes the patient says frankly that she is unhappy with the result and you have to agree that her feeling is warranted. The remark may be, "it looks as if nothing had ever been done." There are some relationships that adversity cements and I remember one particular patient for whom this was true. She wanted me to do the surgery again and I did it but even with a re-do, the nature of her facial laxity was such that two years later she looked about the same as she had prior to ever having had the operation. At that point, I felt that my surgical intervention in her case was over.

A great advantage for the surgeon who has his own operating room is that the patient is not charged for subsequent touch-ups. This is not possible if one depends on the facilities of a hospital. Managing these financial obligations of the patient who has to have corrective surgery and has to pay for it personally can be "sticky." Perhaps it is wise to have in the original consent form a statement that the patient having cosmetic surgery is responsible not only for the bills at the time of the operation but also bills for the management of any complications that might result. As a matter of principle I do not charge the patient, but the hospital certainly will.

In summary, the major areas in managing the dissatisfied patient are: distorting reality, blaming the patient, inhibiting the patient's anger and fear and increasing guilt, remaining distant or unavailable, failing to consult, trying to jettison the patient, and not structuring a sound treatment plan with the avoidance of premature corrective surgery.

It is perhaps too simple to state that we should treat the patient as we ourselves would want to be treated.

So great is the ill-will among physicians that each denies honour and praise to the other. They would harm a patient and even kill him than grant a colleague his meed of praise.
PARACELSUS
Die grosse Wundarznei (Book II)

THE DISSATISFIED PATIENT AND YOU AS CONSULTANT.   The consultant who sees a patient with an unfavorable result arising from the work of another surgeon is in a singular position to do considerable good or irrevocable harm [56, 154]. Although in this situation, as in any other medical circumstance, the first obligation is to the patient, one can also help the other doctor.

The first step is to obtain as objective a history as possible. Exclamations of disbelief at the patient's story or the other surgeon's behavior should be assiduously avoided. Usually the patient who is angry and distraught gives a too brief history because he or she wishes something done immediately to correct the undesirable result. Since the operation the patient has relived the unfortunate surgical events thousands of times and may be impatient with the consultant for laboriously trying to fit together the sequence. However, securing a full account is crucial.

Typical statements from unhappy individuals are:

"I went to him because he is supposedly tops in his field. How could he have done this?"

"He never told me this could happen. I was in and out of his office—one, two, three."

"He was there to take my money before he operated. But afterward, I could never get near him. I'd call his office and his secretary would say 'He is seeing patients now. He'll be in touch with you.' But he never called back."

As part of the history, it is advisable to ask patients about their general health and their professional and family life, as one would do if that person had come to you initially. What are his or her relations with spouse, parents, and employer? Is there a psychiatric history? Is the patient now abnormally depressed? How has he or she reacted to previous operations?

The physical examination is usually less of a problem than the history. The patient is almost eager to show the scars that "shouldn't be there," the breasts that "don't match," the nose that "looks awful," the tendon graft that "doesn't work." For the consultant, the pitfall is being so absorbed in the local problem that he or she neglects the patient in totality. The consultant might fail to notice, for example, how scars have healed from past trauma or other surgery; or he or she might not detect systemic disease, such as malfunctioning thyroid. During examination it is best, once again, to avoid comments, articulated or not, such as a low whistle, a stare of surprise, or an "Oh my" headshake. The patient will be alert to any sign of how bad the consultant feels the problem is or how badly he or she thinks the other surgeon performed.

The patient should be asked to return to the consulting room for a proper discussion with both of you seated. Most likely the patient resents the other doctor's not spending enough time with him or her and would not want another opinion on the fly, no matter how impressive the consultant's credentials.

Now comes the most difficult part of the consultation—literally "the moment of truth." My experience has been that it is best to give the patient as honest an appraisal of his or her problem as possible but to do so with warmth and empathy. It is helpful to begin simply. "Mrs. Palmer, as you know, you have had a breast reduction and your problem is that the scars are more noticeable than you want. It is true also, as you have said, that the breasts are not symmetrical. I am sure that for you and Dr. _____ this has been very distressing since we both know that he would have wanted the best result for you." Having structured the problem, one can proceed to the treatment, which, for the patient, is the most important derivative of the consultation. "Now, Mrs. Palmer, we would all agree that we have to decide what to do. Looking backward is not productive and can be very upsetting." Although there are times when a consultant should defer his or her opinion because the other surgeon has requested it, generally it is wise to give a candid but not condemning evaluation at the time the patient is seen. Patients fear conspiracy among doctors: that we will protect the worst actions of the most incompetent to maintain the solidarity of our guild. Unfortunately, in some instances this is not mere paranoia.

It is important to ask the patient's permission before getting in touch with the other physician, unless the other physician has sent that patient specifically to the present consultant. We have no legal or ethical right to breach confidentiality without such consent. Aside from the legal implications, we will lose our credibility if the patient feels that there has been communication without his or her knowledge, and we will have rendered ourselves less effective in our helping role. Even if the patient gives permission but is in our office without the other surgeon's knowledge, there is significant strain upon the consultant, especially if the other doctor is a close friend. The strain is even greater if the patient does not give permission for such contact. Usually, however, the patient will agree to it if you can make him or her realize that it is in his or her best interests to obtain as much information as possible about the entire medical course. If the patient is suspicious and has grudgingly consented, one may telephone the doctor in the patient's presence. This three-way discussion, besides allowing an exchange of facts and thoughts, does much to defuse an unpleasantly explosive situation.

Like the denouement in a well-constructed novel, the consultation should result in a plan of management. For all concerned, it is better to look forward in hope than backward in anger.

A practical matter must soon be resolved: Who is now responsible for the patient's future care? Sometimes the patient will settle the matter by refusing to return to the former doctor. Frequently the other surgeon has arranged the consultation and, of course, will continue the care.

I do not believe that it is wise medically or correct ethically to force patients to return to a doctor they no longer trust or like even though their attitudes might be unjustly founded. The plastic surgeon who consults, and we all do, must be willing to assume responsibility in these difficult situations, as we routinely do for the patient coming to us from surgeons not in our specialty. The fear of being unpopular or embroiled in a lawsuit should not lead us to avoid aiding the patient. As a practical matter, a patient whom you, as the second or third surgeon, refuse to treat, is more likely to seek redress by going to an attorney.

At some point in the consultation the truth should be reiterated: that in surgery, as in all of life, perfection is the aim, rarely the attainment; that in our own practice unfavorable results and frank complications have occurred and we can easily sympathize with both the patient and the other doctor. Some may call this being charitable; it is, in fact, being realistic. The patient must realize that our efforts will not magically rectify a difficult problem. In indicating the limitations of our own procedures, we must at the same time not make the patient feel that he or she has been so deformed as to be beyond help. This is the most delicate balance to achieve. Occasionally it does happen that nothing further can be done. The patient must understand this reality, but his or her comprehension and adaptation will be enhanced by a general explanation rather than a cold, peremptory presentation.

The consultant should be sufficiently mature not to use the patient's misery to denigrate a colleague or to plump his or her own ego. The golden rule is eminently pertinent here. Since all who operate are bound to have failures, rejoicing secretly in someone else's poor result is childish and short-sighted. Beware the boomerang!

A consultant who is able to help a patient in trouble also helps a family and a colleague. There are few situations in medicine that demand greater sense and sensibility but yield more satisfaction.

THE DIFFICULT PATIENT

The difficult patient is different from the just described dissatisfied patient, who is a step beyond. With the difficult patient, things are not going right but they have not yet gone wrong, at least ultimately. You both have a chance.

When you are having increasing difficulty in relating to or in helping a patient with his or her problem, the direct approach is the best [80]. Tell the patient that you are concerned about the breakdown in communication. "You seem to be upset. Are you angry with me?" The patient's response will largely dictate the subsequent dialogue, which you should try to keep from becoming a petulant confrontation. After this airing, things generally improve. Occasionally a minor irritation has incited and perpetrated a patient's unhappiness and hostility. The complaint may be completely justified, or the patient may have misinterpreted your words or actions or both. Frequently the issue is less important than the emotions it has aroused. The cause fades while the effect stays. However, that you have shown concern and have made an effort to be friendly and helpful may be all the evidence a patient needs to regain confidence in your commitment to his or her well-being. Sometimes the relationship that has been stunted may now grow into something vigorous and satisfying to you both. Crucial to recovery is the patient's cooperation, or better still, his or her participation. Some ideas of what an intelligent human being can do to help himself may be found in Cousins' book, *The Anatomy of an Illness as Perceived by the Patient* [31]. Passive assent is preferable to active rebellion, but creative participation is the ideal.

While the last is rare, it is worth striving for; but it requires a skillful doctor with humility to recognize personal limitations and the potential of the patient.

I recall a patient who two days after a parotid tumor (pleomorphic adenoma) was removed was being "difficult," according to the nurses, although ostensibly everything was going very well. She complained about the nurses "never being around" when she wanted them. She said that the residents "didn't really care" about her and that I "just breezed in and breezed out" of her room. In actuality, her comment about me was probably true. As she became more testy, I became more distant—just the opposite of what I should have done. Finally, I asked her why she seemed to be always in a bad mood when things were going along very well with respect to her surgery. I did not have to probe deeply; her immediate response was, "It's my son. He told me before I came in for surgery that he was getting married and I can't stand the girl." After this catharsis, her mood in the hospital improved although the situation at home remained the same. Of course, the psychodynamics of all "difficult patients" are not that transparent. Moreover, in many instances, you are the cause of the problem— not something external to you such as a son's poor choice of your patient's daughter-in-law.

Recently I had to cancel a patient's facelift because I was ill for a day. She was furious. "Why me? In all my planning, I never considered the possibility that you would get sick," she moaned. She wanted me to cancel someone later in the week to get her on the schedule. I refused, despite numerous calls from her and her husband. We told her that she would be scheduled when the next opening was available—in a few weeks. On questioning the patient in more detail about why she was so distraught and so anxious to have the surgery as soon as possible, she told me that her father was dying in a nursing home and her mother was in the same condition at her house. She had hired a nurse for the week of her scheduled operation. Furthermore, her son was to be married in four weeks and she wanted to look "normal" for that occasion. I was more sympathetic with her plight and she was more reasonable, although I still detected smoldering resentment. Predictably, she was excessively conscious about each bruise and bump following the operation; that it went well was truly fortunate for us both.

Sometimes we consider a patient to be "difficult" when we think he or she should be grateful. Doctors, like most human beings, appreciate thanks for their efforts and the human animal is not alone in this quest for gratification. A good retriever revels in the satisfaction of his owner. An occasional patient whom we have seen through severe illness not only appears ungrateful but hostile and distant after health is restored. This behavior may make the physician feel rejected, unloved, and even angry. The explanation may be that the patient not only has a disquieting memory of the illness and hospitalization but also is ashamed of having been exposed, mind and body, for all to see. He is like the person who under the ease of alcohol tells all the night before but then shies away from his confidant the next morning.

Few human beings can accept their vulnerability and the patient who stalwartly refuses to look backward in gratitude may be asking you to reconsider her or him now as a normal human being in a normal setting. Frequently, these patients may thank you several months later, when they might admit that they had a difficult time in reintegrating. Some have said, "Sorry I was so difficult."

THE DISAPPEARING PATIENT: GET READY, GET SET—GONE!
About once a year, a patient in the hospital for elective surgery, such as a breast reconstruction or a facelift, will decide against it and will ask to be discharged. Your response logically should be to determine why she has apparently changed her mind (in my experience, the patients who suddenly reverse their resolve have been women). Unless a specific incident, such as rudeness from a nurse or resident, has prompted her departure, you should support her decision and not try to dissuade her from it. While you may be surprised by the suddenness of her action, you probably will have already observed signs of the patient's indecision even during the initial consultation: Perhaps she has asked you to tell her whether or not she should have the operation, or telephoned you frequently to pose innumerable questions more for assurance than for information. Characteristically, she may have changed her admission

date several times, to the exasperation of your secretary. By leaving the hospital, the patient has done both of you a favor. If she was that much in conflict over her procedure, she would likely have been dissatisfied with her result.

Canceling an operation the night before is not solely the patient's privilege. Obviously you would do it for medical reasons, such as an upper respiratory infection or an electrocardiographic abnormality. Occasionally, however, you will have second thoughts about what you could accomplish for him or her. On your preoperative visit, you may get the uncomfortable impression that the patient expects more than you can deliver. It is better to part company then rather than later under more unpleasant circumstances. Although it would have been much better not to have scheduled or admitted the patient, never proceed with an operation that is doomed from the outset. No schedule is inviolable. It takes a strong person to halt the machinery. Be flexible enough to reverse the field or abandon it. If you terminate a patient's stay preoperatively, you should pay for any costs that that person has incurred since you should have come to that conclusion before the patient was hospitalized. Naturally, if the patient is discharged because of a previously unsuspected medical problem, then you do not have to assume financial responsibility. What I am referring to here is eleventh-hour recognition of an error in patient selection.

THE PATIENT IN THE EMERGENCY ROOM

The patient dies while the physician sleeps.
WILLIAM SHAKESPEARE
The Rape of Lucrece

Few would argue against the principle that every physician should respond to an emergency with promptness, courtesy, and competence [26]. Yet, the reality is different. Herbert Spencer, the nineteenth-century English philosopher, believed that the course of most human lives in our society is absurd: As a youth, one is poor and finally when he accumulates enough money, he is too old to enjoy it. Far better for the young to have it initially. Spencer would have seen his desideratum fulfilled in the procedure for staffing most emergency rooms. They are the realm of the under-40 generation. Surgeons just out of residency still revel in their accelerated pace and strain to be summoned in this initial phase of practice. Emergency room patients keep the young surgeon's skills sharpened and the rent paid. The new patient is a certain antidepressant for the beginning doctor. After a few years, elective surgery will increase and emergency calls decrease, for several reasons. Other younger doctors will have joined the staff; they have supplanted you in the "needy" category. Peers refer to peers; the distancing factor of aging is such that residents and nurses feel more comfortable in a medical interchange with those of their own age, provided, of course, that he or she is competent. Another reason for receiving fewer emergency calls as you get older is that you like them less and want them less. No longer do you respond with the same alacrity—instead of a whistle of delight, you emit a groan of reluctance. You may say something such as "O.K., I'll get there when I can."

With more years in practice, the type of work you do will also change. You may now be treating an occasional patient with a hand injury or a facial fracture. This is not the place to discuss how this evolution affects the image or influence of plastic and reconstructive surgery in your community, with your colleagues and the public, or the balance of power with other specialties, such as otolaryngology, oral surgery, and orthopedics.

At meetings, some surgeons in their late 60s state they still "cover" emergency rooms. If they are in a city, the reality is that although they may retain their place on the roster, someone younger is usually assuming call. There is a macho factor here, relating to their wanting not only to prove to themselves and others that they are energetic and as dedicated as before, but also to deny that they are doing esthetic rather than traumatic surgery—much like the medical student who does not want anyone to know that he or she is studying.

Whatever your decision about the emergency ward, your position must be unambiguous. If you are truly on call, then be available and gladly enter the fray.

In watching myself and others in the emergency room, I have noted some common errors in the care of patients.

1. *Being too brusque and abrupt.* Admittedly, any emergency call is unexpected and disrupts your schedule. Conveying your displeasure to patients increases their agony and guilt since they probably are blaming themselves for the accident. Most people are aware that some doctors "do not come out for emergencies"; they will greatly appreciate your efforts and the image of our profession will get a needed boost. A kind word and a sympathetic attitude will help the relationship with the patient who is frightened and in pain and who may not have called you. In an emergency, the circumstances do not permit the gradual forging of a bond between patient and doctor. Yet, in plastic surgery, as one colleague commented, "The emergency room may be a nuisance but it makes you feel like a doctor." Imagine yourself or a loved one with facial injuries and you may then realize that for the patient, the surgeon is the only agent of hope.

2. *Neglecting associated injuries.* This error arises from being too intent on the local problem to the exclusion of other sites of trauma, particularly brain, spinal cord, chest, pelvis, or lower extremities. Facial lacerations are so compelling that even trained personnel may forego the usual workup to treat the obvious. You may be told that the patient is "fine except for the face." Examine the patient yourself before accepting anyone's appraisal.

Another mistake is the frequent omission in the chart of a statement concerning the patient's vision in the instance of facial injury. This basic evaluation should be made. Aside from the medical importance for the patient, it may have legal consequences for you.

3. *Giving excessive reassurance about the eventual scar.* During the repair of a facial laceration, it is tempting to overdo your reassurance of the patient with regard to the scarring that so concerns him or her. In more temperate moments, the plastic surgeon would be the first to state that wound healing is due only partly to the method of suturing. The patient may remember your prediction and if the scar is worse than anticipated, you will receive the blame if you have been too optimistic. For documentation, photograph the patient before you begin your repair.

It is not your fault that the patient was injured; assume the responsibility only for careful care, not for the final result. Paré knew better. "I treat; God heals."

THE PATIENT WITH WHOM YOU ARE TERMINATING
YOUR CARE BUT NOT YOUR CARING

At some point, a surgeon can do no more for a well patient with respect to treatment, operative or otherwise, although he or she may continue to be the patient's friend and medical adviser. Usually, the expectations and perceptions of the surgeon and the patient are similar and terminating is natural and pleasurable. However, some finish under less favorable circumstances. In those situations, the patient is dissatisfied and angry, but, paradoxically, as Shakespeare wrote, "Parting is such sweet sorrow." "Sorrow" because you have not pleased the patient but "sweet" because his or her departure has freed you even though it has been a rejection. But you do have the obligation to tell the patient, preferably in your office and also by letter, that you are no longer responsible for his or her care. You might succeed in referring that person to another source of help. Or things may have deteriorated to the point that your every suggestion is an anathema. Certainly if the patient has a suspected or proven malignancy, these steps of proper termination are mandatory, not just for protecting yourself legally but for ensuring the patient's well-being.

Even the patient who thinks you have mismanaged his or her treatment will grudgingly recognize your attempts to do what a good physician should. And you will also be preserving the tradition of medicine, no mean objective.

Sometimes a patient will not want to leave. He or she may still want more to be done, more than you can do or wish to do. Reluctance on the part of the surgeon may not be due to technical limitations but rather to concern that the patient is becoming surgically dependent and cannot break away to get on with life. The patient should not base his or her future on the results of a minor scar revision, for example. Many surgeons during a long course of treating the patient may insist that the person resume work before the next stage, as a means of rehabilitation.

Occasionally, the patient is ready to quit but the surgeon is relentless. Excessively perfectionistic, he or she subtly or openly coerces the patient into additional procedures to optimize the result. The patient's face has become an extension of the surgeon and his or her handiwork.

When to let well enough alone is a difficult judgment in all of life, not just within the realm of plastic and reconstructive surgery. As the surgeon, if you believe that the patient should be satisfied with what you consider an acceptable result that you cannot further improve, then gently suggest that he consult someone else. Frequently, another surgeon will be able to offer a better solution and, if not, his opinion will confirm yours and the patient may end the quest. If, however, the patient still has difficulty in living with the results, psychotherapy may be beneficial. The problem may be getting the patient to follow this advice. Family support may be crucial to convince the patient of its value.

There are other circumstances in which a patient may refuse to leave. For male surgeons, it is usually a female patient, perhaps of a hysterical personality type. She may not be the sole cause of this situation. Consciously or unconsciously, you may have been emitting signals that she has been eager to recognize. You must emphasize to the patient that you are happy she has done so well and seems satisfied with your care as a physician. Now she no longer needs your medical service but others do. You must be strong enough to recognize that you have the power and the responsibility to terminate the relationship that has gone from the therapeutic to the amorous. Medicine is complicated enough and should be sufficiently challenging without these other ingredients, which serve not only to worsen the interaction between the doctor and the patient but ultimately to make the patient (and usually the doctor) more unhappy.

Perhaps the ancient Indian practitioners were correct in their admonition: "A physician is forbidden to take anything but cooked rice from the hands of a woman." A danger is the Pygmalion complex [96, 97]. You recall the Greek legend about Pygmalion, a sculptor, who carved a beautiful ivory statue of a woman and then fell in love with it. In answer to his prayers, Aphrodite transformed his work of art into a living woman, whom Pygmalion married. Some female patients and some plastic surgeons have this primitive fantasy, which does not take much to nurture to a dangerous degree. With the entry of more women into medicine, one might postulate that the same problems will arise but that there will be a sexual reversal of this classic theme.

Under certain circumstances, you may have little recourse but to terminate unilaterally your relationship with the patient. Among the situations that may justify the discharge of a patient are abusive treatment of you by the patient; continued refusal to pay bills when you have used all reasonable means to collect; when the disease from which the patient suffers is foreign to your expertise; repeated failure of the patient to follow your advice; excessive consultations by the patient with other physicians without your knowledge and consent; incompatibility of personalities; when you desire to limit your practice; and when you retire [25]. You have the obligation, however, to notify the patient in writing (registered mail) of the fact that you are discontinuing his or her treatment and to make an effort to supply an appropriate substitute. You should also try to communicate with the patient's family and friends to be sure they understand the reason for your action so that you cannot be accused of abandoning the patient.

THE DYING PATIENT

The noise of carriages and carts, the rattle of wheels, the cries of men and boys, all the busy sounds of a mighty multitude instinct with life and occupation, blended into one deep murmur, floated into the room . . . the breaking of the billows of the restless sea of life that rolled heavily on, without. Melancholy sounds to a quiet listener at any time; how melancholy to the watcher by the bed of death!
CHARLES DICKENS
Pickwick Papers (Chap. XLIV)

I was born to a lifetime of dying.
HENRY DE MONTHERLANT
Chaos and Night

We are but skin about a wind, with muscles clenched against mortality.
DJUNA BARNES

The majority of patients in the care of most plastic surgeons are not in the end stage of disease. Exceptions are those with advanced melanoma or malignancy of the head and neck. The dying patient presents for the average plastic surgeon an unusual therapeutic situation. But no physician, even someone whose specialty is the terminal patient, should become so inured or detached that the demise of his or her patient is seen as a routine event, without significance and tragedy for someone.

This is not the place nor do I have the experience to present observations such as those of Kübler-Ross [85, 86] and others [148] who have documented in the dying patient a sequence of denial and isolation, anger, bargaining ("If only I can live until my son graduates."), depression, and finally acceptance. The point I wish to make is not to let the patient feel grotesque and isolated. Do not allow yourself to be fearful of contact with him or her. The issue is often not so much how a patient can accept the situation but how well the doctor does.

The fact that you do not have a cure does not render you useless [148]. This is the time to be a physician, not just a doctor. No matter how many times you treat a dying patient, terminal illness never becomes easy but why should we expect it to be? To help the patient and yourself and to make your efforts more effective, gather the support of the patient's family, good friends, the nurses, the oncologist, other patients, the radiotherapist, the family doctor, and the clergy, if appropriate for that person. However, with those others to help, resist the temptation to run away yourself. If the patient considers you to be his or her doctor for that particular time in life, do not disappoint him or her. Your ability to bring comfort to this person and his or her family will be good preparation for the next dying patient, perhaps ultimately for your own demise, unpleasant as it is to contemplate. The family also can benefit from support groups, which are increasingly available.

In *A Physician Faces Cancer in Himself*, Sanes [126], whose learning experience unfortunately came firsthand, offered advice about dealing with a presumably incurable patient, someone with disseminate cancer. He stressed the value of "competence, compassion, and communication"—desiderata for relating to any patient, not just the very ill. His advice was: Be available; be punctual; take time ("one minute sitting down is worth five standing up when speaking to a patient or a member of his family"); be open but not casual, objective but not cold, warm and concerned; avoid interruptions (e.g., telephone calls); be truthful and honest within the limits of available knowledge; use simple, understandable language, not medical terminology or jargon; avoid expressing your thoughts and emotions in nonverbal forms that may upset the patient or family; if the patient has cancer, say the word and specify the type of cancer; use a printed sheet or a diagram to help get the message across; do not try to give all the information at once; listen to the questions that family members ask and then answer them to the best of your ability; see that the family gets information and advice about nonmedical problems that may arise as a result of the patient's cancer; give the family your telephone number; assure them that you will not abandon the patient and them for the duration of the illness and beyond. Be prepared to repeat in the future some of what you have said during the first interview and to expand upon it; acquaint the family about new developments, including changes in treatment and reasons for them; keep your promises to the patient and family; do not get angry if asked about a new proven or unproven treatment or procedure reported in the press or elsewhere and whether it could be applicable to the patient's case; do not get angry if a friend of the family intervenes; provide encouragement and support and preserve hope as far as possible.

While cheerfulness is desirable, avoid humor that may be decidedly inappropriate and even cruel. Telling jokes to someone who has only a short ration of days improves neither their state of mind nor your image as a physician and friend. Occasionally, you may be using humor as a way of preventing the person from making you deal with the central, hard issues. Remember that the patient wants you to be there; whereas your desire may be to escape.

THE PATIENT AND THE LAW

This heading could be the title of a massive text, but for purposes here, I wish to discuss only a few aspects.

Undoubtedly, malpractice suits would be rare if medical treatment met the expectations of every patient [72]. The reality is different. The fact that most people in the United States believe that anyone can sue anyone else has resulted in the popularity of that indoor sport: going to court. A generation ago, a common saying was, "Go ahead, sue me! It's a free country." Today only a fool would utter such a statement. Since only one side usually wins, not all suits are victorious (or meritorious) and, in the case of physicians, more are acquitted than are found guilty. Presumably, the better the doctor-patient relationship, the less the likelihood of legal action. Even with the best possible performance by a physician, however, an occasional patient will feel injured, wronged, overcharged, or undergratified. The only way to avoid a malpractice suit against you professionally is to relinquish being a doctor, a course so defensive and distasteful that few physicians, unless close to retirement, will take it. Just as cars have bumpers, so do doctors have malpractice insurance. No matter how carefully you select your patients and perform their surgery, no one is immune from an occasional legal tussle with an unhappy patient. Although it would be unwise to live in constant fear of a lawsuit, it is reasonable to take some measures to prevent a court action. Throughout this book I have tried to indicate those situations in which the behavior of a doctor can negatively affect his or her relationship with the patient. At any time but especially at certain strategic junctures (such as the operating room), the interaction can deteriorate. Proper patient selection, competent treatment, and careful record keeping are important practices in helping you avoid the halls of justice. The trick is to be careful without becoming compulsive and paranoid in dealing with patients. One would not wish to become a fretful physician, viewing each patient as potentially malevolent. Gone would be the pleasure of medicine and the delights of doctoring.

In the section on the dissatisfied patient, I have discussed specific measures to restore a crumbling alliance. Every human activity has its dangers and being a patient or a doctor is no exception. Even though the incidence of lawsuits has increased, it still is not an ordinary event for most physicians, although the concern with its possible occurrence is pervasive. Most doctors have a strong sense of its presence in the background—an unfailing source of disquiet.

Gorney [68] has given 10 commandments for minimizing risks of suits for malpractice.

1. Thou shalt attempt to understand thy patient.
2. Thou shalt listen to thy patient.
3. Thou shalt not "sell" thy trade.
4. Thou shalt treat thy patient as thyself.
5. Thou shalt own up to thy mistakes immediately.
6. Thou shalt not operate when in doubt.
7. Thou shalt not commit thyself to guarantees—stated or implied.
8. Thou shalt seek consultation when in doubt.
9. Thou shalt speak no evil of thy colleague.
10. Thou shalt eschew arrogance.

These dicta, which deserve not only to be remembered but to be followed, have been discussed in various contexts in this book, especially in relation to informing the patient and informed consent. To Gorney's rules should be added that of being cautious when attempting a new and unproven procedure and that of carefully reviewing the nursing notes daily as well as any report by a consultant [72].

Let us consider a few medical situations relating to the law.

Should you treat lawyers or their close family in elective circumstances? This question is not so absurd as it may at first seem since some plastic surgeons refuse to render therapy to attorneys or their spouses and children. The reason ostensibly is to avoid a lawsuit, but I believe that the major cause is generalized hostility toward the legal profession and its practitioners. This behavior on the part of physicians is puerile and is as unreasonable as what they consider the behavior of lawyers to be. Regarding all attorneys as enemies is paranoid and harmful thinking that will certainly create or reinforce their antipathy toward medicine. In my experience, lawyers and their families—perhaps they are conscious of the traditional antagonism between the professions—try to be exemplary patients. In fact, their understanding of the limitations of the operative procedure and the impossibility of guaranteeing results facilitates rapport. Of course, with any group— lawyers, teachers, manual laborers—some individuals are difficult patients and because of their personality traits, not their occupations, should be rejected for elective surgery. As physicians, we know that treating other doctors may not be an easy chore, although the risk of one doctor's suing another is much less than that of a patient outside the medical profession.

Should you treat a patient who has sued a physician? Again, you must make your decision on the basis of the individual patient. Your first responsibility is toward the patient who, in fact, may have been justified in instituting legal proceedings and you, the physician, should not add to his or her misery by abstaining from rendering proper care. But, just as that patient has a right to sue, so you have a right not to treat in circumstances other than an emergency.

Should you assiduously avoid involvement in any malpractice suit on behalf of any defendant or any plaintiff? The obvious answer is that you must decide according to the specific case. The reality is that testifying against another doctor will be an uncomfortable experience and may cause you considerable enmity. But you also have the responsibility of monitoring your profession. If the object of each attorney were to establish the truth, as is supposedly the aim of the judge and the courtroom, your position would be much easier. However, as one distinguished plaintiff attorney told me, "Most lawyers want to win their case and will do so in any way. They justify their actions by saying that it is for the good of their client. Truth is a happy by-product but do not be surprised if it gets lost in the scuffle."

Some physicians refuse to go to court even to present testimony on behalf of a patient whom they have treated after facial trauma. They do not consider that presentation of their findings and management is part of their duty to the patient. Some doctors even request that the patient sign a form releasing them from court appearances. Although one cannot say that such an attitude is right or wrong, it does seem to me to be somewhat extreme. Perhaps those doctors are wiser than I but I do feel that a patient deserves my recounting his or her physical examination and treatment, either by letter (preferably) or in court should the need arise. Often this information can be obtained by a deposition in your office.

Like most human beings, physicians will fight for some things and not for others. I do not like to wait in line at a restaurant but I will for a good movie. Some physicians will exert themselves in the legal arena whereas they will not in order to write a paper or do research. One thing is certain: Whatever you decide, be prepared.

4. The Plastic Surgeon:
Personality, Priorities, and Performance

I observe the phisician *with the same diligence, as hee the* disease.
JOHN DONNE
Devotions (1603)

From inability to let well alone: from too much zeal for what is new and contempt for what is old; from putting knowledge before wisdom; science before art and cleverness before commonsense; from treating patients as cases and from making the cure of the disease more grievous than its endurance, Good Lord, deliver us.
SIR ROBERT HUTCHINSON
(Cited in *Proc. R. Soc. Med.* 64:1038, 1971)

Throughout this book I have described and discussed the interaction of patient and plastic surgeon. I have given numerous instances of when and how the bonding can be thwarted, strengthened, or weakened. In this chapter my purpose is to focus once again on the surgeon but not to the exclusion of the patient.

The Early Stage
Shakespeare described seven ages of man. The reader will excuse my presenting only three ages of the surgeon. The earliest encompasses the first years after residency, when new surgeons, to be successful, must *unlearn* part of their training. Not every facet of a residency is optimal for future performance. The frenzied pace of most training programs forces residents to survive by rushing through tasks and by mastering shortcuts.

For example, making rounds and not sitting down in a patient's room is standard procedure. In fact, a recognized ploy is to see patients so early in the morning that they will be too groggy to respond meaningfully to the routine question, "How are you today?" Rare is the surgeon who actually sits by the bedside and lets the patient talk without imparting an impression of having one foot already out the door. Most patients feel guilty about being a nuisance to their harried doctor. From guilt, it is an easy step to anger at the surgeon for not listening and not caring. These sentiments on the part of the patient are usually justified. We surgeons would do well to remember the advice of our great progenitor, Theodore Billroth [14]. "The patient longs for the doctor's daily visits; it is the event upon which all his thoughts and emotions turn. The physician can do all he has to do with speed and precision, but he must never appear to be in a hurry, and never absentminded." The dictum "Stop, look, and listen" has validity beyond the railroad crossing.

Another important difference after residency relates to responsibility. In most training programs, only the chief resident is truly responsible for his or her decisions, and even then, someone is available to share the grief: the head of the service or the staff member attending for that month. Some chief residents, more than others, delegate to those junior members tasks and obligations that should be theirs, such as talking to the patient and the family about the coming operation. But on that last day in June, when school is out, when students shed their residence status and cross the Rubicon, it becomes necessary to adapt to the new circumstances of assuming more responsibility for their actions, unless they have chosen a protected environment as a subaltern. Not every young surgeon can accommodate easily to these new demands and expectations. Patients are now more likely to consider him or her as their principal physician during the course of their treatment. Although the young practitioner can get advice, he or she cannot hide in the shadows. An irate patient may forgive a resident who is learning but not a full-fledged surgeon who should know. This accountability has its benefits: The person who can be the target of blame can also receive praise. People will eventually recognize a job well done; the surgeon's status, material and otherwise, will improve. Having helped others, the young practitioner at the same time has helped him- or herself. The ancient Greeks recognized the importance of what psychologists today call positive reinforcement: "When there is no reward, there is no excellence."

But the path of the young surgeon (or any doctor) is not one of only pleasures. There are pitfalls as well.

Early in practice surgeons may extend their indications to operate in order to get experience, build a following, and pay the rent. ("A virgin surgeon needs no urgin'.") As residents, they were rewarded for scouting the wards for cases. "The more the better" could be their epithet. Those who supervise residents know that the problem is more to restrain them from the operating room than to urge them toward it. From June, when they finish their training, to a week later in July when they begin their practice, they not unexpectedly continue their accustomed behavior. Professional and financial pressures are greater now than during residency. A young surgeon who unwisely commits himself or herself to unwieldy fiscal burdens, such as a grand house with a grander mortgage, is liable to become more indiscriminate, consciously and unconsciously, in patient selection. As the feeling of entitlement increases, the sense of proportion decreases. For the young surgeon and spouse, luxuries become necessities. Perhaps they are following the advice of Oscar Wilde, "Take care of the luxuries; the necessities will take care of themselves." Unfortunately, that epigram may augur poorly for the patient, who may become grist for that prodigal surgeon's mill. Many human beings in other areas of life, not just plastic surgeons, have the problem of keeping their ambition and hedonism in moderation and their ideals in focus.

Although I have emphasized some negative aspects of the beginner in practice, there are strongly positive features of that stage in professional life. To begin with the most obvious: New plastic surgeons are young enough to be energetic and enthusiastic. Furthermore, they probably have learned many things that an older plastic surgeon does not know: at the moment, for example, microsurgical technique for free flap transfer and the many varieties and uses of musculocutaneous flaps. Another significant advantage is that they have more time to devote to being doctors. Because they have fewer patients, they theoretically can remain longer with each one. Since their total professional commitments are less onerous than are those of someone who is established, they can engage in patient care with less fragmentation. In short, young plastic surgeons have tremendous potential, but unless they are careful they may fall victim to what Alfred North Whitehead observed,

"Youth is wasted on youth." They must remember that they have chosen a profession in which service is still expected. Helping others is the most certain way of bringing success to themselves and, incidentally, favor to their profession.

The Middle Stage

Heaven defend me from a busy doctor.
WELSH PROVERB

After having been in practice 10 to 20 years, the plastic surgeon is probably in the full flush of his or her profession. Better known and more in demand, he or she now has the problem not of getting patients but of treating them properly. Great is the temptation to operate on more patients than would be wise because of a feeling of invincibility, that one's experience has been so extensive and one's skills so remarkable that nothing can possibly go wrong. This type of thinking is an occupational disease associated with upward surgical mobility. To manage the large influx of patients, the surgeon may add systems and personnel that may hinder his or her connection with the patient. Enlarging one's office, taking on one or more associates—all are part of the picture of growing bigger but not necessarily better. Where is that careful and considerate doctor of yore? As we rake in the money, we may also be raking in the patients, as if they were leaves. In some offices, for example, the receptionist may greet the patient, a secretary may take information (address, age, occupation, insurance coverage) and may even obtain a history. A computer may even do the questioning or the patient may be asked to fill out a questionnaire. Later, a technician may take blood and ask for a urine sample or do an electrocardiogram. During this process, the patient may justifiably wonder, "Is there a doctor in the house?" In the name of efficiency, the system has been fabricated presumably so the doctor can treat more people more competently. The paradox is that although the doctor gains in time, the quality of his or her relationship with the patient may suffer. The patient is receiving adequate care but inadequate caring. Even in this age of acceleration, the interaction between physician and patient, in order to be worthwhile, must take time. In the "olden days" (as my children refer to my youth, but actually, long before), the doctor-patient relationship was strong possibly because almost everything else was weak. Hospitals were nonexistent or primitive; nursing, pharmacology, and the knowledge of disease and the body mechanisms were comparatively rudimentary; surgery was the last resort and the most dangerous. The doctor, his skills, and his presence were the cornerstone of medicine. Now with more support, such as better nursing, better surgery, and better trained colleagues, the individual doctor has become only part of the medical picture. He or she must fight to maintain position on the stage. Crowding but helping the doctor and patient are platoons of people—secretaries, receptionists, technicians, orderlies, other doctors, social workers, dietitians, respiratory-occupational-physical therapists—and this list is incomplete. The permeation of urban culture into almost every area of the United States and most Western societies has diluted the sense of mutual responsibility. Commitments of family members to each other are sadly tenuous and unenthusiastic. The young wish to live alone and leave the old to die alone. "Doing your own thing" and "taking care of numero uno" are trite phrases for a virulent disease that has infected medicine and has weakened the special bonding between doctor and patient. But nostalgia for what was is a futile indulgence since that era is gone forever. Even if we could have it back, would we want it? Would we wish to be once again without skilled anesthesia, antibiotics, vaccines?

To return to the busy doctor's office of today, one might question whether taking the blood, obtaining an electrocardiogram, and removing sutures help the relationship between doctor and patient. Although it is impossible to designate a specific act as "the one" that a doctor should do, there is the reality of the therapeutic ambience. "The laying on of hands," ancient in traces, still is a potent emotional derivative for the patient and the physician. Physical contact with the patient—shaking hands, an arm around the shoulder, taking out stitches—brings the patient and doctor closer together. Consider the banal matter of dressings [104]. For centuries, much has been written about their many functions and attributes; rarely mentioned, however, is that the act of applying, removing, or changing a dressing is an important focal point in the doctor-patient relationship and has ritualistic significance. The patient is usually more aware of the subtleties involved than is the physician. Respect for the dressing is respect for the patient and your craft.

Is the dressing neat, comfortable, and effective? Does it annoy the patient by repeatedly falling off? In the hospital, do you change the dressing initially or do you manage to avoid that task by relegating it to a nurse or a resident? Do you give the impression to the patient and the staff that caring for the dressing is really beneath your position or beyond your time? If you do change the dressing, is it with gentleness and calmness? Or do you rush into the patient's room, abruptly turn on the lights, pull down the bedclothes, and rip off the dressing without a prelude of conversation or explanation? Are you careful about your aseptic technique when indicated? Do you then use sterile gloves? (It is interesting how many patients seem to remember more about Lister's precepts than do their doctors.) Do you have all your supplies ready or do you have to interrupt the procedure several times to get what you need? A disorganized, heavy-handed performance in changing a dressing would logically leave the patient wondering how carefully you did the operation.

Surgeons who see more patients than their skills and time can encompass will take the easy ways. Something has to go and, unfortunately, it may be not just their dressings but their standards. The concern, compassion, and competence that brought them to the rung of the "successful" may soon be jettisoned. No longer are they what they were or what they should be. Because labels stick for a long time, a few years may have to pass before one's halo is noticeably faded. By then, the way back may be impossible because there is too much relearning to do.

Admittedly, some patients, comparatively few, do not mind that the doctor has spent minimal time with them [44]. They are content to bathe in the reflected narcissism of their doctor—to delight in the physician's aura of success, as if magically his or her status will protect them against illness or guarantee the success of an operation. These patients find consolation in the elaborate "setup" of their doctor's office, which, for them, is evidence of favor with the gods.

For the discerning patient, however, the doctor has become a medical businessperson, marketing charm and competence without truly caring, still perhaps able to focus skills on the procedure but not capable of sustaining important medical duties. When a complication occurs, the doctor may instinctively hide behind secretaries, nurses, and assistants, who now become two-legged barriers to the patient. Now "all that glitters is not gold"; the parade, once resplendent, has turned into a dismal spectacle. Little wonder that with the scene soured, the patient may contemplate legal recourse.

The predicament of today's doctor in mid-career is the complexity and range of necessary activity—from office to home, and back and forth from one hospital to the next; the financial realities of maintaining a place of practice as well as a residence and family; the voraciousness of the paper tiger—unending forms and correspondence; the medicolegal spectre and the need to stay informed and to deal successfully and sympathetically, if possible, with thousands of patients, some on an emergency basis. Having more, doing more, but enjoying it less could be the slogan of our age. Busy doctors bolting from one commitment to another fit too well into today's tableau. In those air-conditioned cars, do they enjoy life as doctors or as human beings more than did their predecessors who visited their patients in horse-drawn buggies? Although individually we cannot do much to change our times, we can do something to modify our schedule. We must learn to protect ourselves from the superabundance of stimuli: noise, media, telephones, insurance forms, meaningless committee work.

How many patients can we see and manage optimally? When the "successful" plastic surgeon begins to make mistakes or feels like a short-order cook, then it is time to pull back although it would have been better to have done so before. The management of success is often more difficult than its acquisition.

Physicians have another problem. We are not like the painter who can discard a shoddy canvas. A mistake for us is also a mistake for somebody else, with possible lethal consequences. That Ted Williams once batted over .400 was astounding for a ballplayer but not good enough for a physician and patient.

Adding to the perplexity of maintaining the "human touch" with those who should be our intimates is the fact of specialization. Within the specialty of plastic surgery, there has been subspecialization. Fewer surgeons are doing a wide range of plastic and reconstructive surgery. Although many might complain about this trend, few can deny it. The phenomenon is related not only to the complexity of medicine and to the availability of more plastic surgeons, but also to the medicolegal climate in our country. Venturing beyond one's skills is not only dangerous for the patient but for ourselves from a malpractice standpoint.

A surgeon who repeats one procedure more often becomes increasingly adept at that procedure and less sure in other undertakings. This cycle reinforces the trend to doing more in a narrow range. Furthermore, a conscious choice to treat what is more financially rewarding will provide another incentive to restrict one's focus. The longer a surgeon is in practice, the more limited his or her spectrum. Soon comes the point when he or she can no longer do well or easily all the procedures that were familiar at the end of residency. In addition, new procedures will evolve for which he or she perhaps can never be trained: for example, microsurgical transfer of tissue and craniofacial surgery. The reality is that where one puts one's energies and maintains a high profile, there is the focal point of patient referral. Someone who gives numerous lectures on head and neck surgery is unlikely to receive referrals for hypospadias repair or for breast augmentation.

The danger of extreme specialization is the likelihood of our becoming technicians rather than remaining plastic surgeons or physicians, and there is the hazard—subtle at first, but pronounced later—of having arrested growth. By doing less and less more and more, doctors will only be able to do less later. They may be priming themselves for mental and spiritual obsolescence. If one has been so unwise and unlucky as to be known for only one procedure, which one does to the exclusion of others, what will happen if it should go out of style—like the mastoid operation of years ago? Will that surgeon have the will and the breadth to re-tread his or her cerebral hemispheres?

A few words about the operation itself, since the plastic surgeon in this mid-career stage will be doing the greatest number of procedures. As we know but like to forget, the operating room may be the arena for spectacular mistakes [55]. A poorly planned or poorly performed operation can be devastating for the patient as well as for the surgeon. The young surgeon makes errors through ignorance and inexperience; the older surgeon errs from carelessness.

Although it is true that bad preoperative and postoperative management can ruin a good operation, only infrequently can a bad operation be transformed into a good one by bedside attention. This is particularly the case in plastic and reconstructive surgery, in which results depend directly upon excellent technique. When the surgeon carries out the procedure in the operating room, it should not be for the first time. The operation should have been done in the mind's eye before, perhaps in the office but certainly in the 12 hours prior to operation, if the case is elective. The design of the flap, the type of immobilization, the availability of blood and proper equipment—considerations of this sort should not be left to happenstance. The ability to ad lib may lend a virtuoso quality to our field but it should never replace tactical thinking. No operation is truly minor, but thinking that it may be is too common among busy, established surgeons, who have earned the treacherous label "successful."

If the patient is in satisfactory condition, no operation should be terminated until it has been done as well as possible. Boredom, fatigue, or the pressing schedule of an overcommitted surgeon should not compromise standards. A result that looks just fair at operation will generally look worse in the office. If a final glance discloses a remediable fault, we should not be reluctant to heed our assessment. A few more minutes can make a startling difference. Time spent then is more worthwhile than apologies and explanations later. Stitches are not sacred; they should be removed and replaced until the desired result is achieved. Michelangelo wisely commented, "Trivials make perfection but perfection is not trivial."

During the operation, the surgeon must never lapse into a cavalier and complacent attitude, but must be attentive to many things, including possible breaks in asepsis. You must check all solutions before using them, and communicate with the anesthesiologist about vital signs and changes in head and body position. At the end of the case, take the time to assess the result objectively; do not let your efforts and energies peter out and trust your reputation to gloss over imperfections. The great operation you might have done last week or two hours ago is irrelevant. It is what you are doing now that counts, for that patient presently in your care.

Concluding the case with the operation is a common folly, observed more among older surgeons than those just beginning practice. In reality, the operation is not finished until the patient has been discharged from the surgeon's care. The hit-and-run technique has no place in surgery. Concern for the patient and his or her problems should not fade from consciousness as soon as the surgeon has applied the dressing (or is he or she too busy to do it or to supervise it?). Careful observation, detailed orders, and clear instructions are obviously critical. Those of us who are blessed with residents should not abrogate our responsibility. We should know, for example, when the patient has pain or some other complaint. We should also be fully aware of the patient's medications, vital signs, and laboratory data. Our standards should not go down with the setting sun. If a dressing or splint warrants removal, it should be done as quickly at night as during the day. The "wait for the morning" attitude may be effective for growing crocuses but not for managing patients.

Another frequent error, discussed earlier in this book, is the attempt to be the bionic surgeon—know all, do all. If a situation presents problems beyond our usual ken, we should be quick to utilize consultants *before* the patient asks or a tragedy eventuates—not just to keep clean medicolegally but, more important, to ensure the patient the best treatment. Those who consult or refer early seldom need to repent later.

Another fault of many surgeons, particularly those with crowded schedules, is to follow up with a non–follow-up. Surgeons who fail to observe their patients long enough and carefully enough will lose a valuable chance to learn and to improve [58]. In contrast, he who believes in extended, thorough observation will behold many things, sometimes wondrous, occasionally painful, always instructive. A year later the revised scar that initially looked so disappointing will have improved miraculously. This being a hard world, the reverse is also true. The rhinoplasty that appeared "perfect" at six months can end up with many imperfections. It is always tempting to quit while ahead: to discharge the facelift patient, for example, when she is rejuvenated and grateful but only for a few months after surgery. If we truly wish to better our performance and to know our patients' reactions to their operations, we should follow them closely and objectively for a few years. During this time we must be genuinely committed to learning; we must not fit new facts into old impressions.

Every surgeon must beware of the sinister saboteur of good deeds—fatigue. An operation is a series of interdigitating sequential acts, whose quality depends upon the soma and psyche of the surgeon, as well as those of the patient. This aspect of the doctor-patient relationship has been discussed before. The point for emphasis is that the overworked, overstressed surgeon does him- or herself little good and may do the patient considerable harm [71]. It would seem logical for us to try to keep fit physically and emotionally for our daily performance. Athletes do and their errors, though disappointing to spectators, rarely kill anyone. Patients, in fact, are very much aware of the health and habits of their doctors. Many patients in the hospital have said to me on afternoon rounds, "Get a good night's sleep, doctor." Or, even more explicit, "No partying tonight," with a nervous laugh. The statement that I am a teetotaler may provide reassurance if I am believed.

The Last Stage

The young man knows the rules, but the old man knows the exceptions.
OLIVER WENDELL HOLMES
The Young Practitioner in *Medical Essays*

When I was young, patients were afraid of me; now that I am old, I am afraid of patients.
JOHANN PETER FRANK
(Quoted by F. H. Garrison in *Bull. N.Y. Acad. Med.* 5:157, 1929)

The surgeon has attained seniority, with its privileges: for example, sitting in the front row at rounds, calling the heads of services by their first names, getting desirable operating time. While not yet Dr. Chips, he may be already the topic of anecdotes among residents and nurses. He has become a father and even a grandfather figure sooner than he had expected. Each July he sees others starting as he did 25 to 35 years ago. "The race will be over too soon," he muses. "I am almost the same age as my old chief when he retired." Thoughts of retirement are replacing those of achievement. From his Olympian perch he experiences a new calmness when he views the hurly-burly below. Though grateful for no longer having to shove, he misses, nevertheless, the scent and sweat of the fray. "That is for the young," he consoles himself. More with his intellect than with his emotions, he tries to accept nature's cycle: youth replacing the elderly until they in turn must go. If the senior surgeon is wise, he will ease the way for youth or, at least, not try to impede its march. Fighting the inevitable will demean him and his colleagues will remember him as he was at the end rather than as he had been during the previous three decades. Most of us have seen or heard of older surgeons trying to keep someone from opening a practice in the same city or blocking his referrals or denying him operating room time. These acts are foolish and ultimately futile; they arise from the bitterness and insecurity of knowing that soon he must depart from the scene; the hard questions are when and how.

A surgeon's manual skills are his or her professional and economic survival. For the older surgeon, these may have deteriorated to a degree that is noticeable—a fact that embarrasses him and endangers others. In the operating room, he is under easy scrutiny. Lapses in performance are more obvious more quickly to more people than they would be in a private office or in the practice of other specialties such as dermatology, psychiatry, infectious disease, neurology, and internal medicine. A bad hand tremor appearing in a sexagenarian is as strong circumstantial evidence of aging as, in Thoreau's words, finding "a trout in the milk."

Many hospitals have a mandatory age for taking away operating room privileges. For an elderly surgeon who no longer can use the hospital facilities, an alternative is to build an outpatient unit but this is a major financial and emotional commitment, especially at his age. He may resolve this dilemma by joining an established "surgicenter" that is run usually by those younger whom hopefully he has not alienated. The essence of being a surgeon is performing operations. The older surgeon, like the old bull at mating time, may try to prove his virility surgically. He may undertake procedures that are beyond his capacity. How disastrous the consequences can be is exemplified by the life of the once-great German surgeon, Ferdinand Sauerbruch, who overstayed his time, to the detriment of himself and the death of others [142].

The older surgeon is usually not so creative as he once was. He may have to settle for having his name appear at the end of a list of authors for whom he has provided money and laboratory space. Whereas once he attracted attention because of his accomplishments, he may now maintain the center of the stage through intimidation. Adding to his problems may be the shameful ingratitude of younger surgeons, some of whom expect instant success and when it is not forthcoming, blame the senior surgeon.

The tradition of those older instructing those younger for the benefit of the patient has been one of the most important reasons for the survival of medicine. Competition in the marketplace should not absolve those older from sharing knowledge with those younger, nor those younger from respecting their immediate predecessors. This is a lot to expect in our current society, which is notably deficient in its homage to the elderly. Witness the plight of aging parents. Realistically, also, the senior surgeon has also to contend with waning vigor. Nabokov [101] described himself as follows: "Each man as he approaches his sixties, and sometimes even before, goes through a crisis not only of feeling old, but of being afraid of old age, afraid of seeing his powers decline . . . . Old age is a succession of renunciations. It's not so much the fear of the end, but the fear that the end comes in an unpleasant way."

The older surgeon may dread retirement because during his busy professional career he may not have accrued enough interests to sustain him when he is not thinking or doing plastic surgery 18 hours a day (and dreaming of it the other six). As he sees the scramble around him, he may think wistfully of the truth of the French proverb, "If youth knew; if old age could."

The last stage or any segment of a career does not exist by itself, independent of the vicissitudes of the personal life: family, friends (or lack of them), health, achievements, failures, joys, disappointments. Rare is a life that is uncomplicated, a straight, level line without unexpected peaks and troughs. As the ancient philosophers observed, the only constant is flux, a situation that relentlessly demands adaptation for survival. These processes and complexities of living need only acknowledgment here but not repetition since others have described them well already [130, 144].

Parthian Shots

After reading this book, one might ask the question that a visiting English surgeon put to me at the end of a day at my office and at the hospital, "Is all this patient care really necessary?" Compared to England, doctors in America, he thought, spent inordinate time with their patients. In his country, he observed that the patient expects less and probably gets less but likely does not appreciate the difference. The last part of the statement is yet to be documented but studies have shown that nonoperative professional time expended per patient is less in the British Isles than in the United States [34]. Also in England as on the Continent, doctors are more likely authoritarian and the patient, more compliant and, overtly, less questioning. In the breast clinic at the Beth Israel Hospital in Boston, for example, in addition to physicians, we have nurses and social workers (and psychiatrists readily available) to talk with the patient about her feelings concerning the lump in her breast, even when she has been told that it is benign and there is no need for a biopsy. One might question whether having a psychological avenue stimulates traffic: Are we, in fact, eliciting more emotions than is good for the patient or even more than might have existed had not the clinic been so psychologically oriented? It may not only be the case that if less is offered, less is expected but, as my English colleague suggested, less may actually be all that the patient requires. We lack cross-cultural studies to supply the needed data.

An apparent paradox is that in the United States, where patients receive so much in comparison to those in other countries, they desire even more, and, more frequently than patients anywhere else, they will go to court if they believe that they have been abused. In the background is the lawyer, whose presence, though vexing and worrisome to the physician, has undoubtedly up-graded the rights of patients and the performance of doctors. It has also been a stimulus to give detailed explanations and explicit in-structions to the patient, perhaps to a degree that is excessive and unnecessary, at least according to English standards.

Although differences exist in the doctor-patient relationship among technologically advanced countries, they may be in-significant in comparison with the universals, such as concern, compassion, and competence—qualities that positively affect most persons, be they sick or well [152]. Admittedly, changes in the social and economic environment of medicine may create obsta-cles between patient and physician, but it is unlikely that there will be an interdiction against skill and empathy from the doctor and appreciation from the patient. The importance of health and of those who help to ensure it guarantees that doctoring will not be-come humdrum and detached as are the routines in the post office. My optimism arises from the fact that the doctor-patient relation-ship has remained remarkably intact despite the buffetings of in-numerable social changes through many centuries.

A colleague supposedly commented, "When patients go to a plastic surgeon, they want to know only two things: can he do it and how much will it cost?" The tenet of this book is that most patients want and deserve more, as would we if we were patients. Providing care without caring is like comparing food capsules to a gourmet meal; the former may provide the calories with a dull efficiency but without any enjoyment. The matter of pleasure and satisfaction is not a trivial consideration. In the long run (and is not a medical career like a marathon?) we, the plastic surgeons, will continue to wither on our professional vine unless we extend ourselves to be more than vendors of services, dispensers of a narrow skill.

If, indeed, Dr. Francis Peabody's dictum [112] is correct, and I believe it is—that "the secret of the care of the patient is caring for the patient"—then how do we promote it or teach it? In fact, can we or should we?

That we should seems undeniable if we believe in the value of kindness in human relations and if we recognize that we live not by bread alone. The more difficult question is how to achieve "caring." I realize with temerity that I have strayed from my office to someone else's pulpit but, at the risk of sermonizing, I wish to offer some thoughts that are not original. To foster concern in human beings for one another is still the primary challenge. The golden rule, honored by words, lies tarnished from disuse. If more noble reasons fail to spur humans to help each other, then perhaps a stimulus more base in the hierarchy of motivation may succeed. Forgive a surgeon's pragmatism, but we who walk upright and possess prehensile thumbs must be taught and must learn that it is in our best self-interest not to be totally selfish. Internalizing the precept is not synonymous with acting in accordance with it. How apt the Italian proverb, "Between the saying and the doing lies the breadth of the sea."

Now back to the office. After 12 harried hours of doctoring, when we look in the mirror, where is the concerned medical student of yesteryear? Somewhere below the concretions of fatigue is a vestige. Diversion and sleep will usually provide that crucial ingredient that enables us to reenter the medical arena. There are, however, some doctors who always place their convenience and needs before the plight of their patients [153]. For those physicians, I recommend forced caring: that is, consciously exerting oneself to care even though you and the patient may recognize the attempt is not spontaneous. With time, it might become so but even if it never achieves that status, your efforts will be appreciated.

The quality of trying, at least, even though the emotion or action is not automatic, has to do with what some have termed ego strength or what others have called courage or grit. It is indispensable to win ball games, to save marriages, and to help patients.

In Camus's *The Stranger* [22], Meursault is condemned because he "does not play the game" and ultimately is judged guilty largely because of the damaging evidence that he had not wept at his mother's funeral. In Camus's words,

A much more accurate idea of a character . . . will emerge if one asks just *how* Meursault doesn't play the game. The reply is a simple one: he refuses to lie. To lie is not only to say what isn't true. It is also and above all, to say *more* than is true, and, as far as the human heart is concerned, to express more than one feels. This is what we all do, every day, to simplify life. He says what he is, he refuses to hide his feelings, and immediately society feels threatened.

In the instance of the doctor and the patient, each would *be* threatened if the other did not do some role playing: saying or acting according to each other's expectations. Camus's antihero ultimately loses his life because of his verbal reluctance and his unwillingness to "play the game." In the practice of medicine, the patient would become the casualty of our gratifying only our own needs and our own feelings all the time.

As physicians, though we may empathize with someone who is ill, the synchrony of our sentiments is only periodic, not continuous. Even then, we really do not experience what hurts and threatens a patient. The Portuguese say, "Only the one with the scar feels it." How rare the physician who named the condition "Christmas disease," in honor of the child first shown to lack clotting factor IX! This act on the part of the doctor is unique, since almost all eponyms glorify those who identify a malady rather than those who have to bear it.

In *The Patients,* Thorwald [143] presents recollections by individuals who underwent pioneering operations for failing organs, such as heart, lung, and kidney. These were momentous surgical events with obvious heroes and heroines; yet the commonplace crises are epochs in the lives of any patient and his or her family: Ever present are risk, pain, fear, and uncertainty. Whenever I become ill, fortunately rarely, and then only with the "flu," I glimpse the dark world of patients. My uneasy sensations, even thousandfold, do not approximate those of the truly sick. Yet, from that brief episode, I am conscious of being a better physician;

unfortunately, I confess, my uplifted state lasts just a few weeks; than I slide back into my usual patterns of doctoring, where I am on the comfortable outside looking in. This distance from the patient is not all bad; it allows us to be objective in our work and to continue without being engulfed by sorrow or revulsion. Yet, as Alan Alda [1], *M.A.S.H.*'s Hawkeye, said to the graduating class at Columbia College of Physicians and Surgeons, "You've had to toughen yourself to death. From your first autopsy when you may have been sick, or cried, or just been numb, you've had to inure yourself to death in order to be useful to the living. But I hope in the process you haven't done too good a job of burying that part of you that hurts and is afraid."

As human beings, in our daily lives we usually place the "hows" before the "whys." We are not comfortable trying to resolve for ourselves existential issues. But a patient who is ill is forced to contemplate the monumental questions of death, purpose, meaning—while we, as physicians, at the bedside, are busily fixing the body parts.

Renewal

You, the plastic surgeon, probably came of age to care for patients independently when you were 33. After another 33 years, your professional life would be nearing its end. In those three decades, you probably will have operated upon more than 20,000 patients and will have consulted on at least two or three times that number—equal to a good-sized city's population. Your memory will be stronger for patients for whom things went spectacularly right or dramatically wrong. For the great majority, where help was wanted and given, few traces may remain in your mind; yet those patients likely recall more about that encounter than   do. Although you intervene for a relatively brief period in the life of that person, you have the opportunity to do considerable harm or good. The impact of your treatment may resound throughout the remainder of that patient's life. In that interaction, you both have the opportunity to broaden your lives by at least one new relationship. While it is true that like every human being, you may not remain static psychologically, physiologically, or chronologically, from where you sit you are the relatively constant feature in the tableau of patient and physician. The succession of patients is your reason professionally for being. Yet, most blessings on this planet are diluted and this is no exception. The need to turn out the work as well as the passage of years tends to erode enthusiasm. Recall the excitement of your first patient in practice: You tingled for involvement and felt the pleasure of exercising your skills, of helping someone, and of sensing gratitude in return. But after 20, 12, or even 2 years in practice, you experience satisfactions differently: The highs are not so high. However, it would be unfortunate if the pleasures of doctoring belonged only to the novitiate. They are there also for the seasoned clinician, the old campaigner. His problem, however, is to rekindle the dampened fires of his enthusiasm. Ralph Waldo Emerson observed, "Nothing great was ever achieved without enthusiasm." But "great" need not describe only superachievements in medicine: the discovery of the circulation of blood, the importance of asepsis, or the existence of hormones. To be a good doctor to each patient is no trivial accomplishment. Let him who doubts the value of a good physician experience a bad one! To doctor daily requires renewal. How to "replenish the well," in Winston Churchill's terms, is the quiet challenge for each of us. To do again with joy what we have done many times before can be a task much harder than the medical problem itself. For some physicians, the next patient is a stimulant; for others, a stone. In the latter instance, the relationship between them will be mechanical and drab, perhaps without a scintilla of satisfaction for either. A story concerns three medieval workmen who were asked what they were doing. The first replied, "I toil from sunup to sundown and all I receive for my pains is a few francs a day." The second answered, "I am glad enough to wheel this wheelbarrow for I have been out of work for many months and I have a family to support." The third replied, "I am building Chartres Cathedral [129]."

Discussion of occupational tedium is usually in reference to factory workers or clerical personnel, but seldom physicians. The public may find it hard to believe that doctors, who have high incomes and considerable respect (and are even the subjects of television series), suffer as do all human beings from boredom and despondency. As a group, physicians are reluctant to express their frustrations. They have trained themselves in stoical tenacity and external imperturbability. *Aequanimitas* has become their byword not only at the bedside of patients but even at their own. Not unexpectedly, in comparison to the general population, physicians have an unusually high incidence of alcohol and drug dependency. Whereas they are the first to suggest treatment for others, they are the last to seek it for themselves when they are abnormally depressed. The advice "Physician heal thyself" is as pertinent today as in biblical times. With most physicians, however, the problem is not illness but ennui. The paradox for doctors is that although they may think that their patients are wearing them down, they may not realize patients are also the means for buoying them up. The interaction between patient and doctor presents an opportunity not just for treatment but for personal growth. Your intervention hopefully has cured or improved the patient's illness or condition. His or her life is better because of you; is yours better because of the patient? In addition to vacations, athletics, hobbies, and religion, the relationship between the patient and the doctor can be a source of renewal, provided that the physician experiences it in a fuller dimension and with more imagination than the patterns of today's living seemingly require and allow. The physician has more than a ringside seat to the human condition. He is as much a participant as is the patient. One who does not feel this communality with that person will ultimately be the loser.

Exploring the uncharted areas of any relationship requires a willingness for adventure. Admittedly, the challenges are less spectacular than those facing Dr. Livingstone, but they are there nevertheless. Because they are less obvious, they are in some ways more difficult. But help is near. "The game is afoot," as Sherlock Holmes would say. Your next patient is waiting.

References

1. Alda, A. Commencement address to Columbia College, New York City, May 16, 1979.
2. Alexander, J. E. Challenges in esthetic plastic surgery. *Plast. Reconstr. Surg.* 52:337, 1973.
3. American Society of Plastic and Reconstructive Surgeons, Inc. Official definition of cosmetic and non-cosmetic surgery. Written communication, November 1979.
4. Aristotle. *Politics*, VII, II. In R. McKeon (ed.), *The Basic Works of Aristotle.* New York: Random House, 1941. P. 1280.
5. Baker, T. J. Patient selection and psychological evaluation. *Clin. Plast. Surg.* 5:3, 1978.
6. Baker, T. J. Complications of rhytidectomy. Presented at 20th Annual Meeting, New England Society of Plastic and Reconstructive Surgeons, Sturbridge, Mass., June 8, 1980.
7. Barber, B. *Informed Consent in Medical Therapy and Research.* New Brunswick, N.J.: Rutgers University Press, 1980.
8. Bass, L. W., and Wolfson, J. H. Professional courtesy is obsolete. *N. Engl. J. Med.* 299:772, 1978.
9. Beale, S., Lisper, H.-O., and Palm, B. A psychological study of patients seeking augmentation mammoplasty. *Br. J. Psychiatry* 136:133, 1980.
10. Bennett, A. E. (ed.). *Communication Between Doctors and Patients.* London: Oxford University Press, 1976.
11. Bennett, G. *Patients and Their Doctors. The Journey Through Medical Care.* London: Bailliére Tindall, 1979.
12. Berenson, B. *Sketch for a Self-Portrait.* New York: Pantheon, 1949. P. 85.
13. Bernstein, N. R. Oral communication, 1980.
14. Billroth, T. *The Medical Sciences in the German Universities. A Study in the History of Civilization.* New York: Macmillan, 1924. P. 154.
15. Bird, B. *Talking with Patients* (2nd ed.). Philadelphia: Lippincott, 1973.
16. Bloom, A. A. Social work and the English language. *Soc. Casework* 61:332, 1980.
17. Blumgart, H. L. Caring for the patient. *N. Engl. J. Med.* 270:449, 1964.
18. Bok, S. *Lying: Moral Choice in Public and Private Life.* New York: Pantheon, 1979.
19. Bosk, C. L. *Forgive and Remember. Managing Medical Failure.* Chicago: University of Chicago Press, 1979.
20. Bosk, C. L. Occupational rituals in patient management. *N. Engl. J. Med.* 303:71, 1980.
21. Bower, J. L. Oral communication, 1978.
22. Camus, A. Preface to *The Stranger.* In P. Thrody (ed.), *Lyrical and*

Critical Essays. Translated from French by E. C. Kennedy. New York: Knopf, 1968. Pp. 335–336.

23. Cassileth, B. R., Zupkis, R. V., Sutton-Smith, K., and March, V. Informed consent—why are its goals imperfectly realized? *N. Engl. J. Med.* 302:896, 1980.

24. Cheever, J. The Trouble of Marcie Flint. In *The Stories of John Cheever.* New York: Knopf, 1979. P. 289.

25. Committee on Ethics and Discipline. On terminating the physician-patient relationship. *Mass. Med. Soc. Newsl.* 19:3, 1979.

26. Committee on Trauma, American College of Surgeons. Guidelines for the Patient-Physician Relationship in the Emergency Department. *Bull. Am. Coll. Surg.* 62:15, 1977.

27. Conley, J. J. Introduction to *Complications of Head and Neck Surgery.* Philadelphia: Saunders, 1979. P. 12.

28. Cosman, B. Experience in the argon laser therapy of port wine stains. *Plast. Reconstr. Surg.* 65:119, 1980.

29. Courtiss, E. H., and Goldwyn, R. M. Breast sensation before and after plastic surgery. *Plast. Reconstr. Surg.* 58:1, 1976.

30. Courtiss, E. H., Goldwyn, R. M., and Anastasi, G. W. The fate of breast implants with infection around them. *Plast. Reconstr. Surg.* 63:812, 1979.

31. Cousins, N. *Anatomy of an Illness as Perceived by the Patient: Reflections on Healing and Regeneration.* New York: Norton, 1979.

32. Dicker, R. L., and Syracuse, V. R. *Consultation with a Plastic Surgeon.* Chicago: Nelson-Hall, 1975.

33. DiMatteo, M. R. A social-psychological analysis of physician-patient rapport: Toward a science of the art of medicine. *J. Soc. Issues* 35:12, 1979.

34. Doorey, A. J. The surgical work day in the British Isles. Some observations from a small sample studied in depth. *Arch. Surg.* 114:970, 1976.

35. Drinker, H., Knorr, N. J., and Edgerton, M. T., Jr. Factitious wounds. A psychiatric and surgical dilemma. *Plast. Reconstr. Surg.* 50:458, 1972.

36. du Gard, R. M. *The Thibaults.* New York: Viking Press, 1939.

37. Edgerton, M. T., Jacobson, W. E., and Meyer, E. Surgical-psychiatric study of patients seeking plastic (cosmetic) surgery: Ninety-eight consecutive patients with minimal deformity. *Br. J. Plast. Surg.* 13:136, 1961.

38. Edgerton, M. T., Meyer, E., and Jacobson, W. E. Augmentation mammaplasty. II: Further surgical and psychiatric evaluation. *Plast. Reconstr. Surg.* 27:279, 1961.

39. Edgerton, M. T. Oral communication, 1979.

40. Entralgo, P. L. *Doctor and Patient.* New York: McGraw-Hill, 1969.

41. Ewalt, D. H., et al. Professional courtesy. *Ann. Plast. Surg.* 3:580, 1980.

42. Figueroa, C. Breast reduction—one woman's story. *Woman's Day*, February 20, 1979. P. 40.

43. Fili, W. J. *Face Lifts: Is There One in Your Future?* Broomall, Pa.: Filicon, 1977.

44. Fischl, R. A. The busy physician or, why don't patients understand? *Ann. Plast. Surg.* 3:495, 1979.

45. Fraser, C. On Analysis of Face-to-Face Communication. In A. E. Bennett (ed.), *Communication Between Doctors and Patients.* London: Oxford University Press, 1976. Pp. 7–28.

46. Fredricks, S. Oral communication, 1978.

47. Friday, N. *My Mother, My Self.* New York: Dell, 1977.

48. Furnas, D. W. Operating room mirror for mammaplasty evaluation. *Ann. Plast. Surg.* 3:578, 1979.

49. Gallagher, E. B. The Doctor-Patient Relationship in the Changing Health Scene. Proceedings of an International Conference sponsored by the John E. Fogarty Center for Advanced Study in the Health Sciences, National Institutes of Health. Held at the National Institutes of Health, Bethesda, Md., April 26–28, 1976. Washington, D.C.: U.S. Government Printing Office.

50. Gersuny, R. *Arzt und Patient. Winse für Beide.* Stuttgart: Ferdinand Enke, 1904.

51. Gifford, S. Emotional Attitudes Toward Cosmetic Breast Surgery: Loss and Restitution of the "Ideal Self." In R. M. Goldwyn (ed.), *Plastic and Reconstructive Surgery of the Breast.* Boston: Little, Brown, 1976. Pp. 103–121.

52. Gifford, S. Cosmetic Surgery and Personality Change: A Review and Some Clinical Observations. In R. M. Goldwyn (ed.), *The Unfavorable Result in Plastic Surgery: Avoidance and Treatment.* Boston: Little, Brown, 1972. Pp. 11–33.

53. Goffman, E. *The Presentation of Self in Everyday Life.* Garden City, N.Y.: Doubleday, 1959.

54. Goin, M. K. Psychiatric Considerations. In E. H. Courtiss (ed.), *Aesthetic Surgery Trouble: How to Avoid It and How to Treat It.* St. Louis: Mosby, 1978. Pp. 17–24.

55. Goldwyn, R. M. Ingredients for Failure. In R. M. Goldwyn (ed.), *The Unfavorable Result in Plastic Surgery: Avoidance and Treatment.* Boston: Little, Brown, 1972. Pp. 2–4.

56. Goldwyn, R. M. The Consultant and the Unfavorable Result. In R. M. Goldwyn (ed.), *The Unfavorable Result in Plastic Surgery: Avoidance and Treatment.* Boston: Little, Brown, 1972. Pp. 5–7.

57. Goldwyn, R. M. Operating for the aging face. *Psych. Med.* 3:187, 1972.

58. Goldwyn, R. M. (ed.). *Long-Term Results in Plastic and Reconstructive Surgery.* Boston: Little, Brown, 1980. Vols. 1 and 2.

59. Goldwyn, R. M. Disease is a family affair. *Arch. Surg.* 106:610, 1973.

60. Goldwyn, R. M. Fees. A perspective. *Arch. Surg.* 107:127, 1973.

61. Goldwyn, R. M. High hopes and malpractice. *Arch. Surg.* 111:1042, 1976.

62. Goldwyn, R. M. Patient Selection: The Importance of Being

Cautious. In E. H. Courtiss (ed.), *Aesthetic Surgery Trouble: How to Avoid It and How to Treat It*. St. Louis: Mosby, 1978. Pp. 14–16.

63. Goldwyn, R. M. The Dissatisfied Patient. In D. Gowlian and E. H. Courtiss (eds.), *Symposium on Surgery of the Aging Face*. St. Louis: Mosby, 1978. Vol. 19, pp. 81–84.

64. Goldwyn, R. M. The Woman and Esthetic Surgery. In M. T. Notman and C. C. Nadelson (eds.), *The Woman Patient. Medical and Psychological Interfaces*. I: *Sexual and Reproductive Aspects of Women's Health Care*. New York: Plenum Press, 1978. Pp. 271–280.

65. Goldwyn, R. M., and Kasdon, E. J. The "disappearance" of residual basal cell carcinoma of the skin. *Ann. Plast. Surg.* 1:286, 1978.

66. Goldwyn, R. M. Unexpected bleeding after elective nasal surgery. *Ann. Plast. Surg.* 2:201, 1979.

67. Goldwyn, R. M., and Strome, M. Unsuspected adenoid cystic carcinoma in secondary rhinoplasty. *Ann. Plast. Surg.* 2:338, 1979.

68. Gorney, M. Malpractice. In E. H. Courtiss (ed.), *Aesthetic Surgery Trouble: How to Avoid It and How to Treat It*. St. Louis: Mosby, 1978. Pp. 1–13.

69. Grazer, F. M., and Goldwyn, R. M. Abdominoplasty: Assessed by survey with emphasis on complications. *Plast. Reconstr. Surg.* 59:513, 1977.

70. Grazer, F. M., and Klingbeil, J. R. *Body Image: A Surgical Perspective*. St. Louis: Mosby, 1980.

71. Green, R. C., Jr., Carroll, G. J., and Buxton, W. D. *The Care and Management of the Sick and Incompetent Physician*. Springfield, Ill.: Thomas, 1978.

72. Griggs, J. Avoiding malpractice suits. *Surg. Rounds* 3(No. 5):64, May 1980.

73. Grundner, T. M. On the readability of surgical consent forms. *N. Engl. J. Med.* 302:900, 1980.

74. Gurdin, M. D. Oral communication, 1977.

75. Haug, M. Doctor patient relationships and the older patient. *J. Gerontol.* 34:852, 1979.

76. Hay, G. G., and Heather, B. B. Changes in psychometric test results following cosmetic nasal operations. *Br. J. Psychiatry* 122:89, 1973.

77. Hetter, G. P. Satisfactions and dissatisfactions of patients with augmentation mammaplasty. *Plast. Reconstr. Surg.* 64:151, 1979.

78. Jacobson, W. E., Edgerton, M. T., and Meyer, E. Psychiatric evaluation of male patients seeking cosmetic surgery. *Plast. Reconstr. Surg.* 26:356, 1960.

79. Johnson, D. Doctor talk. *New Republic*, August 18, 1979. Pp. 25–27.

80. Kahan, E. B., and Gaskill, E. B. The "Difficult" Patient: Observations on the Staff-Patient Interaction. In M. T. Notman and C. C. Nadelson (eds.), *The Woman Patient. Medical and Psychological Interfaces*. I: *Sexual and Reproductive Aspects of Women's Health Care*. New York: Plenum Press, 1978. Pp. 257–269.

81. Kalick, S. M.   Aesthetic surgery: How it affects the way patients are perceived by others. *Ann. Plast. Surg.* 2:128, 1979.
82. Kalick, S. M.   Written communication, 1980.
83. Karsh, E.   The Doctor-Patient Relationship Through the Ages. In W. E. Preece (ed.), *Medical and Health Annual.* New York: Encyclopaedia Britannica, 1977.
84. Kaye, B. L.   Rhinoplasty in the older patient. Presented at the 10th Annual Symposium on Aesthetic Plastic Surgery, University of Toronto, Toronto, Ontario, March 28, 1980.
85. Kübler-Ross, E.   *On Death and Dying.* New York: Macmillan, 1969.
86. Kübler-Ross, E.   *Questions and Answers on Death and Dying.* New York: Macmillan, 1974.
87. Kunstler, W. E.   Aesthetic considerations in surgical operations from antiquity to recent times. *Bull. Hist. Med.* 12:27, 1942.
88. Lederer, H. D.   How the Sick View Their World. In E. G. Jaco (ed.), *Patients, Physicians, and Illness. Sourcebook in Behavioral Science and Medicine.* New York: Free Press, 1958. Pp. 247–256.
89. Leff, L.   A Secret of Success: Be Good at Getting Wrinkles Ironed Out. *Wall Street Journal,* November 15, 1979.
90. Ley, P.   Towards Better Doctor-Patient Communications. In A. E. Bennett (ed.), *Communication Between Doctors and Patients.* London: Oxford University Press, 1976. Pp. 77–98.
91. Lipkin, M.   *The Care of Patients: Concepts and Tactics.* New York: Oxford University Press, 1974. Pp. 171–175.
92. Lipp, M. R.   *Respectful Treatment. The Human Side of Medical Care.* Hagerstown, Md.: Harper & Row, 1977.
93. MacGregor, F. C., et al.   *Facial Deformities and Plastic Surgery. A Psychosocial Study.* Springfield, Ill.: Thomas, 1953.
94. MacGregor, F. C.   *Transformation and Identity. The Face and Plastic Surgery.* New York: Quadrangle/Times Books, 1974.
95. Magraw, R. M.   Social and Medical Contracts: Explicit and Implicit. In R. J. Bulger (ed.), *Hippocrates Revisited.* New York: MedCom, 1973. Pp. 148–157.
96. Maltz, M.   *New Faces—New Futures: Rebuilding Character with Plastic Surgery.* New York: R. Smith, 1936.
97. Maltz, M.   *Doctor Pygmalion. The Autobiography of a Plastic Surgeon.* London: Museum Press, 1954.
98. Meyer, E.   Psychiatric Aspects of Plastic Surgery. In J. M. Converse (ed.), *Reconstructive Plastic Surgery* (1st ed.). New York: Saunders, 1964. Vol. 1, pp. 365–383.
99. Morini, S.   Sculpture. What Plastic Surgery Can Do to Give You a Beautiful Bosom. *Vogue,* January 15, 1971. P. 83.
100. Musgrave, R. H., and Garrett, W. S., Jr.   Preoperative Consultation: A Different Concept. In Millard, D. R., Jr. (ed.), *Symposium on Corrective Rhinoplasty.* St. Louis: Mosby, 1976. Pp. 50–55.
101. Nabokov, V.   Quoted in *The New York Times Book Review,* October 24, 1971. P. 22.

102. Nadelson, T.　The Münchausen syndrome. Borderline character features. *Gen. Hosp. Psych.* 1:11, 1979.

103. Noe, J. M., Barsky, S. H., Greer, D. E., and Rosen, S.　Port wine stains and the response to argon laser treatment: Successful treatment and the predictive role of color, age, and biopsy. *Plast. Reconstr. Surg.* 65:130, 1980.

104. Noe, J. M., and Kalish, S.　A New Approach to Wound Dressings. In *Wound Care.* Greenwich, Conn.: Chesebrough-Ponds. Pp. 1–18.

105. Notman, M. T.　A Psychological Consideration, Mastectomy. In M. T. Notman and C. C. Nadelson (eds.), *The Woman Patient. Medical and Psychological Interfaces.* I: *Sexual and Reproductive Aspects of Women's Health Care.* New York: Plenum Press, 1978. Pp. 247–255.

106. Novak, M.　Psychocutaneous medicine: The distrustful patient. *Cutis* 19:362, 1977.

107. Ohlsén, L., Pontén, B., and Hambert, G.　Augmentation mammoplasty: A surgical and psychiatric evaluation of the results. *Ann. Plast. Surg.* 2:42, 1979.

108. Osmond, H.　God and the doctor. *N. Engl. J. Med.* 302:555, 1980.

109. Parsons, T.　Social Structure and Dynamic Process: The Case of Modern Medical Practice. In T. Parsons (ed.), *The Social System.* New York: Free Press, 1951. Pp. 428–479.

110. Parsons, T.　Definitions of Health and Illness in the Light of American Values and Social Structure. In E. G. Jaco (ed.), *Patients, Physicians and Illness. Sourcebook in Behavioral Science and Medicine.* New York: Free Press, 1958. Pp. 165–187.

111. Parsons, T.　The sick role and the role of the physician reconsidered. *Milbank Mem. Fund. Q.* 53:257, 1975.

112. Peabody, F. W.　Care of patient. *J.A.M.A.* 88:877, 1927.

113. Penn, J. G., and Baker, J. L., Jr.　An office-based elective surgical center. *Ann. Plast. Surg.* 4:94, 1980.

114. Phelps, D. B., Buchler, W., and Bostwick, J. A., Jr.　The diagnosis of factitious ulcer of the hand: A case report. *J. Hand Surg.* 2:105, 1977.

115. Rees, T. D.　Selection of Patients. In T. D. Rees and D. Wood-Smith (eds.), *Cosmetic Facial Surgery.* Philadelphia: Saunders, 1973. Pp. 17–26.

116. Rees, T. D.　Written communication, 1980.

117. Rees, T. D.　The Initial Office Consultation. Teaching course of the American Society of Aesthetic Plastic Surgeons, 13th Annual Meeting in Orlando, Fla., May 21, 1980.

118. Rees, T. D.　*Aesthetic Plastic Surgery.* Philadelphia: Saunders, 1980.

119. Reich, J.　The surgery of appearance. Psychological and related aspects. *Med. J. Aust.* 2:5, 1969.

120. Reich, J.　Factors influencing patient satisfaction with the results of esthetic plastic surgery. *Plast. Reconstr. Surg.* 55:5, 1975.

121. Robbe-Grillet, A.　*Jealousy.* In two novels: *Jealousy* and *In the Labyrinth.* Translated by R. Howard. New York: Grove Press, 1965. Pp. 41–42.

122. Rogers, B. O.   The development of aesthetic plastic surgery: A history. *Aesth. Plast. Surg.* 1:3, 1976.
123. Rollin, B.   The Best Years of My Life. *N.Y. Times Magazine*, April 6, 1980. P. 36.
124. Rosenberg, M. L.   *Patients: The Experience of Illness.* Philadelphia: Saunders, 1980.
125. Rudofsky, B.   *The Unfashionable Human Body.* New York: Anchor, 1974.
126. Sanes, S.   *A Physician Faces Cancer in Himself.* Albany: State University of New York Press, 1979. Pp. 40–50, 188–197.
127. Schultz, R. C.   *Outpatient Surgery.* Philadelphia: Lea & Febiger, 1979.
128. Seneca de Beneficiis, VI, 16.   Cited by P. L. Entralgo, *Doctor and Patient.* New York: McGraw-Hill, 1969. P. 7.
129. Shahn, B.   *The Shape of Content.* Cambridge, Mass.: Harvard University Press, 1978. P. 91.
130. Sheehy, G.   *Passages.* New York: Dutton, 1976.
131. Shipley, R. H., O'Donnel, J. M., and Bader, K. F.   Psychosocial effects of cosmetic augmentation mammaplasty. *Aesth. Plast. Surg.* 2:429, 1978.
132. Siegler, M., and Osmond, H.   *Patienthood. The Art of Being a Responsible Patient.* New York: Macmillan, 1979.
133. Sigerist, H. E.   *A History of Medicine.* II: *Early Greek, Hindu, and Persian Medicine.* New York: Oxford University Press, 1961. Pp. 309–310.
134. Sihm, F., Jagd, M., and Pers, M.   Psychological assessment before and after augmentation mammaplasty. *Scand. J. Plast. Reconstr. Surg.* 12:295, 1978.
135. Smith, J. W., and Baker, S. S.   *"Doctor, Make Me Beautiful."* New York: David McKay, 1973.
136. Snyder, M.   The many me's of the self-monitor. *Psych. Today* 13(No. 10):32, March 1980.
137. Sontag, S.   The Double Standard of Aging. *Saturday Review*, September 23, 1972. Pp. 29–38.
138. Sontag, S.   *Illness as Metaphor.* New York: Farrar, Straus, & Giroux, 1978.
139. Spencer, F. C.   The Gibbon Lecture. Competence and compassion: Two qualities of surgical excellence. *Bull. Am. Coll. Surg.* 64:15, 1979.
140. Stallings, J. O., with Moss, T.   *A New You. How Plastic Surgery Can Change Your Life.* New York: Van Nostrand Reinhold, 1977.
141. Thomson, J. A., Jr., Knorr, N. J., and Edgerton, M. T., Jr.   Cosmetic surgery: The psychiatric perspective. *Psychosomatics* 19:7, 1978.
142. Thorwald, J.   *The Dismissal: The Last Days of Ferdinand Sauerbruch.* New York: Pantheon, 1961.
143. Thorwald, J.   *The Patients.* New York: Harcourt Brace Jovanovich, 1971.
144. Vaillant, G. E.   *Adaptation to Life.* Boston: Little, Brown, 1977.

145. Walster, E., Aronson, V., Abrahams, B., et al.   Importance of physical attractiveness in dating behavior. *J. Pers. Soc. Psychol.* 4:508, 1966.
146. Weiss, T. E.   What is hostility? *Phys. East* 1:20, 1979.
147. White, A. G.   The patient sits down: A clinical note. *Psychosom. Med.* 15:256, 1953.
148. White, L. P. (ed.).   Care of patient with fatal illness. *Ann. N.Y. Acad. Sci.* 164:635, 1969.
149. White, R.   Quoted in Honorable intentions. Six ways of looking at a primary care residency. *Harvard Med. Alumni Bull.* 54:11, 1980.
150. Williams, J.   The Initial Office Consultation. Teaching course. The 13th Annual Meeting of the American Society for Aesthetic Plastic Surgery. Orlando, Fla., May 21, 1980.
151. Williams, P., and Harrison, T.   *McIndoe's Army. The Injured Armies Who Faced the World.* London: Pelham, 1979. P. 31.
152. Williams, R. H.   Management of the Sick with Kindness, Compassion, Wisdom, and Efficiency. In R. H. Williams (ed.), *To Live and to Die: When, Why, How.* New York: Springer-Verlag, 1974. Pp. 134–149.
153. Wright, M. R.   Self-perception of the elective surgeon and some patient perception correlates. *Arch. Otolaryngol.* 106:460, 1980.
154. Wright, M. R.   Management of patient dissatisfaction with results of cosmetic procedures. *Arch. Otolaryngol.* 106:466, 1980.
155. Zalon, J., with Block, J. L.   *I Am Whole Again. The Case for Breast Reconstruction After Mastectomy.* New York: Random House, 1978.

Appendix

223

The following are samples of printed material that some surgeons and I give to patients. Undoubtedly other forms and information sheets from other surgeons could have been chosen. My purpose here was not to include everything, but to present examples, which, the reader must remember, represent what these individual surgeons designed to meet their perceived needs and those of their patients. These forms should not be slavishly copied by every surgeon in the expectation that they will perfectly satisfy their requirements or those of their patients. Furthermore, even if the forms should be adequate today, they may not be tomorrow. We must have the flexibility to change our thoughts and actions according to reality. The "reality" is not just medical but personal, social, and legal.

Robert M. Goldwyn, M.D., Inc.

Authorization Form for Excision of Lesions

_____

(Patient's name)

1. I authorize Robert M. Goldwyn, M.D. (the "Doctor") to perform an operation upon me (or my _____)
   to (description of procedure):

2. The nature and effects of the operation, the risks and complications involved, as well as alternative methods of treatment, have been fully explained to me by the Doctor and I understand them.
3. I authorize the Doctor to perform any other procedure that he may deem desirable in attempting to improve the condition stated in paragraph 1 or any unhealthy or unforeseen condition that may be encountered during the operation.
4. I consent to the administration of anesthetics by the Doctor or under the direction of the physician responsible for this service.
5. I understand that the practice of medicine and surgery is not an exact science and that reputable practitioners cannot guarantee results. No guarantee or assurance has been given by the Doctor or anyone else as to the results that may be obtained.
6. I understand that the two sides of the human body are not the same and can never be made the same.
7. For the purpose of advancing medical education, I consent to the admittance of authorized observers to the operating room.
8. I give permission to Robert M. Goldwyn, M.D., Inc. to take still or motion clinical photographs with the understanding that such photographs remain the property of the corporation.

I certify that I have read the above authorization, that the explanations referred to therein were made to my satisfaction, and that I fully understand such explanations and the above authorization.

Signed _____

(Patient or person authorized
to consent for patient)

Date _____

Witness _____

Bernard L. Kaye, M.D., D.M.D.

Nose Surgery Instructions

I. BEFORE YOUR OPERATION

(AVOID SCHEDULING SURGERY DURING MENSTRUAL PERIODS)

Preliminary
1. No aspirin or medicines containing aspirin for four weeks before surgery, since it interferes with normal blood clotting. If needed, use Tylenol instead. (That means NO Alka-Seltzer, Anacin, Ascriptin, BC, Bufferin, Cheracol capsules, Cope, Coricidin, Darvon Compound, Fiorinal, Dristan, Empirin, Excedrin, Midol, Sine-Aid, Sine-Off, Percodan, Stendin, Triaminicin, Vanquish, etc. If in doubt check with us.)
2. Smokers should cut down to three or four cigarettes a day for three days before surgery. Smoking irritates nasal passages and causes coughing, which might bring on a late nosebleed several days after your operation.
3. Report any signs of a cold, infection, boils, or pustules appearing within three weeks before surgery.
4. Arrange for someone to drive you to your home, hotel, or motel after surgery.

Night Before Surgery
Wash your face with Dial or Safeguard soap. Do not cream your face afterward.

Day of Surgery
1. No makeup.
2. *Nothing to eat* for six hours before surgery. May drink small amounts of *clear liquids* (water, black coffee, tea, sodas, etc.) up to three hours before surgery.
3. Do *not* take *medication* of *any kind* (unless instructed by Dr. Kaye). Your preoperative medications will be given to you upon arrival.
4. Wear comfortable, loose-fitting clothes that do not have to be put on over your head.
5. Bring a scarf and sunglasses to wear after your operation.
6. You *must* have someone to drive for you after surgery. On arrival at office, give secretary your driver's name and phone number, as well as address and phone number where you will be the night after surgery.
7. You *must* have someone spend the first night with you. Additional instructions and prescriptions can be given to the person calling for you. Such prescriptions should be filled promptly.

8. If you have any questions before your operation, please call our office weekdays between 9:00 A.M. and 5:00 P.M.

II. AFTER YOUR OPERATION
 1. Bed rest with two pillows for 24 hours.
 2. May go to bathroom with assistance as needed.
 3. Take medications according to instructions on bottle. If taking strong narcotics (i.e., Demerol, Dilaudid) or if other pain medications make you feel "spacey" or drowsy, have someone else give you your medicines according to the proper time intervals. Under such circumstances you could forget and take them too often.
 4. Soft diet requiring little or no chewing. Lots of liquids. Avoid very hot foods or liquids.
 5. *No hot or warm compresses!*
 6. You can expect:
    a. Initial nosebleed for about four hours. Change "drip pad" gauzes under your nose as needed.
    b. Moderate discomfort—use pain medicine (see #3 above).
    c. Swelling and black and blue around your eyes, sometimes more on the second or third day after surgery than the first.
    d. Blood-shot "whites" of your eyes.
 7. Call (396-2816) if you have:
    a. Severe pain not responding to medications.
    b. Prolonged profuse bleeding (soaking more than five drip pads per hour after four hours).
    c. Any other question or problem.
 8. During the first week following surgery:
    a. Restrict talking and walking to a minimum.
    b. Avoid lots of visitors.
    c. Do not bend your head down.
    d. Do not strain to do anything that requires significant effort.
 9. No smoking for seven days after surgery, because it irritates the lining of the nose and causes coughing, both of which could bring on a late nosebleed.
10. No alcohol for 10 days after surgery.
11. No nose drops for 10 days after surgery.
12. Do not blow your nose for two weeks after surgery. After the first week you may gently cleanse your nostrils with a moist Q-tip.
13. You may wash your hair on the third day after surgery (not counting the day of surgery), providing you have someone help you wash it in the *face up* position. *Do not* bend your head forward. You may blow it dry with a warm hand dryer or sit under a cool dryer.

14. You may wear any makeup, providing it does not interfere with the splint or tapes.
15. If you happen to sneeze, it usually causes no harm.
16. Avoid sports and other strenuous activity for four weeks.
17. Avoid prolonged exposure to sun and/or heat for three months to prevent prolonged swelling.
18. Feel free to call on us at any time. We want you to be as comfortable as possible during your healing period.

Office Visits

First: One or two days following surgery if Dr. Kaye thinks it is necessary to see you soon. Otherwise—

Second: Approximately one week after surgery, at which time your nasal splint will be removed and you will be given a lighter tape splint.

Third: Approximately five days later, when your tape splint will be removed. If the stitches have not dissolved, they can be removed at this time.

Additional visits: Will be determined by Dr. Kaye.

John E. Williams, M.D.

Some Facts on Nasal Surgery

To: My Patients

We usually perform surgery to improve the shape and function of the nose in our office surgical unit. The anesthesia consists of heavy sedation, and local infiltration. A packing is placed inside the nose, which numbs the lining; the remainder of the infiltration of the local anesthesia is carried out through this numbed lining. There is very little, if any, pain or discomfort during the operation, and except for headache and a feeling of stuffiness, no real pain in the postoperative period.

Since the operation is done entirely through the nostrils, there will usually be no scars outside the nose. Following the operation, which usually takes just under two hours, a pressure dressing is applied to the eyes to prevent some of the swelling and bruising. The eye bandages may be removed at home the first morning following the operation. Because of this blindfold and sedation, someone must be with you the first night. At the completion of the operation, a light packing is placed inside the nose, and this is removed in the office in 24 to 48 hours. In addition, when the operation is over, a plaster splint is applied to the outside of the nose, in order to hold it in the desired position. This splint is removed in the office on the fifth to seventh day, and must not be removed except in the office.

Most of the swelling and bruising occurs around the eyes since these are the softer structures. The bruising is usually completely gone within seven days, as is a good portion of the swelling. This period of time can be shortened considerably by the use of ice-water compresses to the eyes, two or three times a day for one hour each time.

The nose is a pyramid-shaped structure attached to the face at its base; there is only one direction in which the nose can swell, and that is upward. This creates a strange appearance to the face for at least the first three weeks, and usually makes it appear that the nose was shortened too much. This is often the cause for much concern by patients unless they understand in advance that as swelling subsides the nose will come down and assume a much more natural appearance. This is more apparent to the patient and the patient's family than to strangers, and the patient can usually return to normal social activities in three to four weeks.

There will be an unusual firmness to the tip of the nose due to swelling and reaction to the surgical procedure. This may persist for as long as four to six months and will continue to soften and improve for as long as a full year in some instances. As a general rule, if one can still feel a firmness at the tip of the nose, it can be assumed that there is still considerable swelling present. It is not unusual for a patient to go through a period of depression and extreme worry about the looks of the nose, and it should be remembered that it is impossible to judge the final results of surgery until all of the swelling has subsided.

Patients vary in their rate of healing and reaction to surgery. The integrity and thickness of skin and deeper tissues vary from person to person and, therefore, the exact shape of the nose cannot be predicted 100 percent. In rare instances a small retouch operation may be required to obtain the optimal results desired.

During the first three weeks after surgery, you must avoid bumping the nose and refrain from exercising too much or becoming too hot. These are the things that prolong swelling and cause the nose to bleed. The hair may be shampooed anytime after the nasal splint has been removed, as long as the water is only lukewarm. If a hair dryer is used, the controls should be on the cool setting and not hot.

Preoperative photographs are as important to the plastic surgeon as x rays are to the chest surgeon. These are medical photographs and are not meant to flatter you. You will probably find them harsh and not suitable for framing. However, these photographs are very helpful in planning and performing the nasal operation.

If you have any other questions, be sure to get them answered in advance by me or by my office staff. Most members of my staff have been with me for years and they are thoroughly informed, trained, and able to answer questions that may occur to you. Well-meaning friends are not a good source of information. Find out everything you want to know, as a well-informed patient is a happy one.

Thomas D. Rees, M.D.

*Some Facts for Patients About Cosmetic Facial and Eyelid Surgery**

To: My Patients

You will do yourself a service if you read what follows carefully, for here you will find answers to many of the questions that are most often asked about plastic surgery of the face, neck, and eyelids. Most of these questions are universally asked by patients interested in this type of surgical correction.

The purpose of cosmetic surgery is to make you look as good as it is possible for you to look. It cannot do more than that. If you are expecting a transforming miracle from surgery, you will unquestionably be disappointed. Plastic surgery is a combination of art and science. Surgery is not altogether an exact science, and because some of the factors involved in producing the final result (such as the healing process) are not entirely within the control of either the surgeon or patient, it is impossible to warranty or guarantee results. Surgical results from facial and eyelid plastic surgery, however, are more predictable in some patients than others. This is determined by a number of factors such as the physical condition of the skin, the presence or absence of facial fat, the relative "age" of the skin, the numbers and types of wrinkles present, the underlying bone structure, heredity and hormonal influences, and others.

It is not possible, by surgical operation, to make someone who is over 40 years old look as if he or she is 20 years old or younger! While this may seem obvious, I mention it because some patients through misconceptions or misinformation believe the clock can be turned back in this miraculous fashion. It cannot.

Surgery intended to improve sagging skin or wrinkles necessarily leaves scars. Despite what you may have heard, all surgical scars are permanent and cannot be erased. The job of the plastic surgeon is to place scars in natural lines of the face and eyelids, where they are least noticeable and are more easily camouflaged by makeup or hairstyles. While such scars are permanent, they rarely are noticeable or cause any trouble.

Now for some specific questions.

1. How long will the surgical results last? Plastic surgery of the face, neck, and eyelids retards the aging process and actually slows it up. It "slows down the clock, but does not stop it." It is not a question of a sudden "falling down." How soon you will want or require another operation is highly individualized. I can only speak in averages. In general, the operation of facial and neck lift, which is for the improvement of the jowls along the jawline and the loose skin of

---

*Copyrighted by Thomas D. Rees, M.D.

the neck, may need to be redone in about five to eight years. Some very few patients are encountered who, for one reason or another, age more rapidly so that another operation may be desired in a shorter period of time than five years. Of course there are some who never require it again. The operation to improve or correct "bags" of the eyelids usually lasts longer. In most instances, the pouches beneath the lower lids do not recur. As one grows older the skin becomes looser and redundant and a trim of loose skin may be necessary at a later time. In those patients where there is exceedingly marked aging and excessive skin of the neck, face, and jaw, sometimes (but extremely rarely) it is necessary to perform a second operation within a year to achieve the maximum improvement possible. If this seems to be the situation in your case, I will so inform you in advance.

2. *Is facial surgery considered to be a major operation?* This type of surgery very rarely produces serious complications. It is, however, a surgical procedure, and as such, can be subject to unpredictables. Fortunately these are usually minor and amenable to treatment. These will be discussed with you in detail if you so desire.

3. *Why are preoperative photographs important?* Just as the chest surgeon cannot operate in an intelligent way without x rays of the chest, the plastic surgeon cannot operate on the face or eyelids without medical photographs. These photographs are not meant to flatter you. You probably will find it a harsh photograph unsuitable for framing. The photos will show your face in every detail. This aids greatly in the surgical performance of technical variations in the surgery.

4. *What type of anesthesia is used during the operation?* Either local or general anesthesia can be used, according to preference. I prefer to use a combination of light general anesthesia and local anesthesia, which I find is more comfortable for the patient. This technique permits a light anesthesia. A high level of oxygen is maintained throughout the surgery, which promotes safety. Local anesthesia is preferred by some patients and is completely adequate for this purpose. General anesthesia requires the services of an expert anesthesiologist who charges separately. His fee is explained in the preoperative instructions. Whether you have a local or general anesthesia, in either case there will be no pain during the operation.

5. *How long is the operation?* The actual surgical time may vary, depending on the amount of surgery necessary for each patient. A facelift usually requires about two hours and eyelid surgery one hour.

6. *How long is the hospital stay?* The usual hospital stay is three days. Admission is usually one day prior to the operation at about 2:00 P.M. and discharge time is about 10:00 A.M. the second or third day after surgery. Admission to the hospital may seem unnecessar-

ily early, but is necessary in order to perform the required laboratory work and examinations by the resident surgeon and anesthesiologist. Although the room accommodations are booked well in advance of admission, it may not always be possible to have the accommodation you desire on admission to the hospital. Every attempt on my part will be made to handle this problem to your advantage.

7. *Are bandages applied?* Bandages are applied to the head and neck after a facelift. These are removed 48 hours after surgery. Bandages may or may not be applied to the eyelids for a few hours. Following removal of the bandages, ice compresses are applied to the eyes for several hours. Although this will not prevent all bruising and swelling, it will help to minimize it. After leaving the hospital these ice compresses may be continued at home from time to time, if you find them comfortable. Bandages are applied for several reasons, one being to keep the operated area as immobile as possible; therefore it is also important that telephone calls and visitors be kept to a minimum for the first 48 hours after the operation. But postoperative pain is rare; and whatever discomfort there may be is usually mild, short-lived, and easily handled with routine medication.

8. *When are the stitches removed?* Most eyelid stitches will be removed on the second day after operation. The remainder are removed on the third or fourth day. Some stitches in front of the ears are removed on the sixth or seventh day after a facelift. In most instances, all remaining stitches are removed by the tenth day. Removing stitches is quick and uncomplicated. But you must remain in the New York area for a minimum of 10 days following facial surgery and one week following eyelid surgery so that the removal may be done.

9. *When can makeup be applied?* Eye makeup may usually be applied three days after the removal of the last sutures. This includes mascara, eyeshadow, and artificial eyelashes. Facial makeup can usually be applied by about the tenth day. At this time, you may have to use some type of covering cream if there are still bruises below the eyes. It is important to remove all makeup very thoroughly, using an upward motion, at the end of the day. Oiled eye pads are recommended for the removal of eye makeup. My office staff will provide detailed instructions on makeup during the postoperative period.

10. *When may I get my hair done?* On the fourth day following surgery, you may comb your hair out by using a solution of warm water and a large-toothed comb. Your first shampoo will not be possible until the eighth day following surgery. You may do this yourself or go to a hairdresser who is acquainted with the special procedure of the first hairset after plastic surgery. My office can recommend someone suitable. Rollers may be used, but loosely. A

hair dryer may also be used but at the "comfort zone" (never hot), since at this time you may not have full sensation in the areas operated on. Tinting and coloring usually may be done about three weeks after the operation.

11. Is the hair shaved in preparation for the operation? The hair is not shaved. At the time of surgery, a small margin of hair behind the ears is trimmed where the incision will be. A similar area is trimmed inside the hairline above the ears. Neither area is visible once the hair is combed over the incision.

12. Who takes care of me after surgery? Except over the weekends, you will be visited every day in the hospital by me. If for unforeseen reasons, I am unable to visit you, you will be seen by one of my staff. There is an expert team of associates and assistants always in attendance, who are continuously in touch with me. It is also not possible for me to visit you the night of admission to the hospital. Therefore, it is important that any unresolved questions be discussed prior to admission, if necessary, by a further visit to the office.

13. Who actually performs the operation? I perform all surgery on my patients. I do have assistants who play an active role in your operation by assisting me just as the anesthetist and nurse do. However, the actual operative procedure is performed by me.

14. What happens in the postoperative period? You must remember that before you see the improvement you are expecting you will go through a standard postoperative period in which you will look quite battered and bruised, followed by another temporary period of time when you may look "strange" to yourself. This varies considerably with each individual. When both facial and eyelid surgery are performed together you should set aside three weeks for recovery. At the end of this time most patients are able to appear in public, although the scars may need camouflaging with makeup. In some patients this time may be shortened by a few days and in others a slightly longer period is required. I think you should also bear in mind that in some patients undergoing facial and eyelid surgery, there is a temporary period of slight emotional depression immediately following the surgery, during the period of time when you look your worst. This is quite normal and should not alarm you. It is not easy to look bruised and swollen, particularly when natural expectations are toward improving your appearance. Fortunately this period usually passes rather quickly.

15. Are private nurses available? Although private nursing care is not a necessity, some patients feel happier knowing that someone will be with them after surgery. Some hospitals require the patient to book private nurses at the time of admission. At other hospitals we are able to arrange for nurses in advance. In spite of booking well in advance of surgery, there is no guarantee that nurses will be available because of the critical shortage of such help.

If you have any other questions, be sure to get them answered in advance by me or my office. Many members of my office staff have been with me for years and are thoroughly informed, trained, and able to answer questions that may occur to you. Well-meaning friends are not a good source of information. Find out everything you want to know. A well-informed patient is a happy one.

Robert M. Goldwyn, M.D.

To My Patients After Eyelidplasty

1. Someone should drive you home. Keep dressings wrung out in ice water on your eyes until you arrive home.
2. Get into bed and elevate your head on two pillows. Stay in bed as much as possible for the next 18 hours. For the next 4 nights, sleeping on your back will decrease swelling and discoloration.
3. Continue the ice-water dressings to your eyes day and night for 24 to 36 hours.
4. Expect some pain and oozing from the incisions. You have been given a prescription for pain medicine, which you should take as directed. Avoid aspirin or aspirin-containing compounds. Tylenol can be used in conjunction with or instead of the prescribed medication (unless you are sensitive to it).
5. You will be given Liquifilm Tears after surgery. Instill two drops into each eye three times a day and when you go to sleep at night.
6. *If* you have been asked to use Saran Wrap to cover your eyes at night, cut out a piece in the shape of an eye mask and apply cellophane tape around the edges to keep your eyes moist. This will protect your cornea during the period when you cannot close your lids completely while asleep. Remember that the Saran Wrap goes directly on your eyes only at night without any intervening ice dressings and should be applied after you have put Liquifilm Tears into your eyes at bedtime.
7. The day after operation, you may be up but continue your ice dressings. Avoid housework and lifting anything more than 10 pounds for another week. Do not resume athletics for two weeks. Dark glasses will make your eyes more comfortable when you go outside and will also decrease questions from the curious.
8. You may wash your face with a cloth and soapy water. Do not wash the incisions. Apply petroleum jelly on the incisions to lessen inflammation and itching.
9. Call my office to arrange an appointment for stitch removal. After sutures are out, you may then begin to use makeup but do not apply it to the incisions until 10 days after surgery.
10. It will take a few weeks for the initial swelling and discoloration to subside. There will likely be temporary differences between one eye and the other. Please be patient. Try to avoid comparing them since it will increase your anxiety without helping your healing. During this immediate postoperative phase, never apply heat in any form to your eyes.
11. For sudden or severe pain, excessive bleeding, or any unusual occurrence, call my office immediately (232-7523).

James L. Baker, Jr., M.D., and John G. Penn, M.D.

Patient Instructions for Surgical Breast Enlargement
(Augmentation Mammoplasty)

GENERAL INFORMATION
Cosmetic enlargement of the breasts is done by surgical implanta-
tion of a breast prosthesis (a medical grade silicone bag) placed
behind the breasts between breast and chest wall muscles.

The amount of breast enlargement is a decision that must be
made by the physician, in that only the physician can make an accurate appraisal as to the correct size of implant that a given breast will
accommodate. However, the patient's wishes and desires, if realistic, will be given maximum consideration. The implant is placed
under the breast tissue, so that any future physical examination of
the breasts by a physician will be possible, as well as breast-feeding
of subsequent pregnancies. There is absolutely *no recorded evidence
relating breast enlargement* (with silicone implants) *and breast cancer.*
Silicone impants are made of nontoxic material that is well accepted
by the body and should last a lifetime.

OPERATION
We prefer to do the surgery under local anesthesia as an office procedure. The patient is sedated and the surgery takes approximately
one hour. The patient returns home shortly thereafter.

INCISION
A small incision, approximately two inches in length, is made either
under the breast or in the armpit. This usually heals to a fine-lined
scar by six months.

POST-OPERATION
The patient is restricted to rest at home with *minimal* arm movement, especially during the first 48 hours. There may be some mild
discomfort, swelling and/or discoloration of the breast area for a
short period of time. A regular brassiere is utilized as the final dressing, one cup size larger than the patient now wears.

POSSIBLE COMPLICATIONS
It is sometimes necessary to remove an implant due to an unforeseen complication; however, this is a rarity. Complications such as
bleeding, infection, or changes in sensation, though unusual, can
occur. Firmness of the breast in varying degrees can also occur.

FEE

In compliance with the suggestions adopted by the American Society of Plastic and Reconstructive Surgeons, Inc., it is routine to request that fees for all cosmetic procedures be paid prior to surgery. Insurance will not participate in fee payment for surgical enlargement of the breasts.

BEFORE-SURGERY INSTRUCTIONS

1. *Do not take aspirin or aspirin-containing (salicylates) compounds* for at least two weeks before surgery. You *may* take *Tylenol* (acetaminophen-containing compound) in their place.
2. *You must have your laboratory work completed 7–10 days before surgery.*
3. *Take nothing by mouth on the morning of surgery.* You must completely fast the morning of surgery with *NO* breakfast. *No* coffee and *no* water. If your surgery is in the afternoon, you may have clear liquids up until 8:00 A.M., which may consist of water, black coffee, or tea with sugar if desired (no milk or milk products) or 7-Up.
4. Armpits should be shaved closely two days before surgery. Do not shave the day before surgery and omit deodorants after your last shower. They may be used again beginning the day *after* surgery.
5. Scrub armpits, breast, and chest wall thoroughly (five minutes with Betadine Skin Cleanser, available at your drugstore without prescription) every day for one week before surgery.
6. On the day of surgery, someone must drive you to our office and take you home after surgery. A responsible person must stay with you the first night at least.
7. It is preferable but not necessary to have the surgery performed when the patient is not in the midst of her menstrual cycle. Our scheduling secretary will attempt to work out the timing of the surgery so that this does not conflict.
8. Bring to surgery a new, unused, all-elastic stretch brassiere, one cup size larger than you now wear. (We recommend the Mary Jane brassiere. If you prefer, we have available, at cost, a brassiere designed for postoperative breast patients.)
9. Have your prescriptions filled at least one week before surgery because you will begin taking certain medications before your operation. Instructions will be on each bottle. The *pain* pills prescription must be filled within 48 hours after it is dated.
10. Wear *loose-fitting* clothing that is easy to slip on and off with *minimal* use of your arms and low slip-on shoes: *No* pullover sweaters or high platform shoes.
11. *Do NOT* wear any jewelry the day of your surgery since it will have to be removed for the operation and may be misplaced in

the office. We cannot assume responsibility for these items if they are lost.

AFTER-SURGERY INSTRUCTIONS
1. *Arm movements.* Limit the use of your arms almost entirely for the first two days after surgery and make only *minimal arm movements* for at least the first week after surgery. Do not lift anything heavy or drive a car during that time. The first 48 hours you should rest indoors as much as possible, preferably in a semireclining position. *Do not take aspirin in any form for at least two weeks.*
2. After one week you may resume most normal activities except for such things as tennis, golf, swimming, or strenuous exercise. These activities may be resumed usually by three weeks. Do not lie or sit in direct sunlight or hot outdoor areas for the first two weeks.
3. *Shampoo and hair coloring.* All coiffure procedures can be carried out at any time the patient desires; however, excessive use of the arms necessary for these acts should be limited the first 10 days, so go to the beauty shop.
4. *Showers and baths.* Sponge baths until instructed otherwise by the doctor (usually three to five days post operative).
5. *Social activity.* Social activity should be limited for approximately 10 days after the operation. Excessive arm movements and exercise should be restricted for the first two weeks.
6. Take all antibiotics and other medications as instructed.
7. Someone should stay with you day and night for 48 hours after surgery.
8. Wear the brassiere we put on in surgery until you are seen in the office for your first postoperative visit.
9. *Pain.* You may expect some discomfort for the first several days postoperatively. This will be similar to a muscle pain after strenuous physical activity. As soon as you begin to feel discomfort after you get home, begin taking your pain pills as prescribed—do not wait until the pain is severe.

James L. Baker, Jr., M.D., and John G. Penn, M.D.

Special Consent to Augmentation Mammoplasty or Other Procedure

Patient _____

Date _____ Time _____

1. I hereby authorize _____ and/or associates to perform a surgical operation for increasing the size or shape of the patient's breasts, known as augmentation mammoplasty, on _____
   (Name of patient) or (Myself)
2. The procedure listed in paragraph 1 has been personally explained to me by the above doctors, and I completely understand the nature and consequences of the procedure. The following points, among others, have been specifically made clear:
   a. The operation has been done for several years, but the end results are not, and cannot be determined for a number of years yet to come.
   b. Research indicates that the material implanted in the body does not cause malignancy in human subjects.
   c. There is a possibility that my body may not tolerate these implants, making it necessary to remove the implants. This occurs in a small percentage of cases.
   d. A cyst may form in the area adjacent to the implants, causing fluid accumulation that may require drainage by needle or removal of the implants.
   e. The breasts can become firm (capsule formation and contraction). This condition can be permanent and can cause pain and discomfort.
   f. No guarantee has been given as to size and shape of the breasts. Good results are expected but not guaranteed.
   g. In some patients the margin of the implants can be felt.
   h. The incision will heal with a scar that will be permanent.
   i. Postoperative bleeding may occur around the implant, requiring a second operation for its removal.
   j. After being exposed to cold temperatures (such as swimming in cold water), the breasts may feel cooler than surrounding body tissues.
   k. Pregnancy is not recommended for at least six (6) months after the surgery.
   l. Numbness or hypersensitivity of the nipple may be experienced following surgery.

241

  m. The procedure is subject to the same postoperative compli-
     cations as other surgical procedures.
3. I recognize that, during the course of the operation, unforeseen
   conditions may necessitate additional or different procedures
   than those set forth above. I therefore further authorize and request that the above-named surgeon, his assistants, or his des-
   ignees perform such procedures as are, in his professional
   judgment, necessary and desirable, including, but not limited to,
   procedures involving pathology and radiology. The authority
   granted under this paragraph 3 shall extend to remedying conditions that are not known to the above doctors at the time the
   operation is commenced.
4. I consent to the administration of local anesthesia to be applied
   by or under the direction and supervision of the above doctors,
   with the exception of _____
                          (None or a particular one)
5. I recognize that when general anesthesia is used it presents additional risks over which the above doctors have no control, and I
   agree to discuss the risks of general anesthesia with the anesthesiologist before surgery is performed.
6. I am aware that the practice of medicine and surgery is not an
   exact science, and I acknowledge that no guarantees have been
   made to me as to the results of the operation or procedure.
7. I consent to be photographed before, during, and after the treatment; that these photographs shall be the property of the above
   doctors and may be published in scientific journals and/or shown
   for scientific reasons.
8. I agree to keep the above doctors informed of any change of
   address so that they can notify me of any late findings, and I
   agree to cooperate with the above doctors in my care after surgery until completely discharged.
9. I am not known to be allergic to anything except: (list)

I HAVE READ THE ABOVE CONSENT AND RECEIVED A
COPY OF IT. I FULLY UNDERSTAND THE CONTENTS
OF THE CONSENT AND AUTHORIZE AND REQUEST
THE ABOVE DOCTORS TO PERFORM THIS SURGICAL
PROCEDURE ON ME.

_____   _____
(Witness)   (Patient)

IF PATIENT IS A MINOR, COMPLETE THE FOLLOWING:
Patient is a minor _____ years of age, and we, the under-
signed, are the parents, guardians, or legal representatives of the
patient.

_____   _____
(Witness)   (Parent or legal guardian)

_____   _____
(Witness)   (Parent or legal guardian)

Frederick M. Grazer, M.D.

Consent for Abdominoplasty

Patient _____ Age _____

A.M.
Date _____ Time _____ P.M. Place _____

1. I hereby authorize Dr. Frederick M. Grazer, and whomever he may designate as his assistants, to perform upon _____

   (State name of

   _____ the following operation(s):

   patient or "myself")

   and if any unforeseen condition arises in the course of this operation calling on his judgment for procedures in addition to or different from those now contemplated, I further request and authorize him to do whatever he deems advisable and necessary in the circumstance.

2. I have been informed that the clinical outcome in my case does not only bear a relationship to the nature of the pathology (that is, the condition revealed, disclosed, or discovered by the procedure or procedures), but also bears a relationship to me insofar as there are individual variations of a physiological nature that influence recovery from the above-described procedure and that may or may not predispose to complications (see below). The nature, purpose, and risk of the operation and procedures and possible alternative methods of treatment and the possibility of complications have been explained fully to me. I acknowledge that no guarantee or assurance has been made as to the results that may be obtained.

3. I consent, authorize, and request the administration of such anesthetic or anesthetics as is deemed suitable by the physician-anesthetist who is an independent contractor and consultant. I fully understand that the physician-anesthetist will have full charge of the administration and maintenance of the general anesthetic and that this is an independent function from the operative procedure, and that Dr. Grazer has no responsibility for or direct control over the administration of the general anesthetic during the surgical procedure(s), and I have been fully informed of and understand that my exposure to anesthesia during the operation may result in adverse consequences, such as paralysis, coma or prolonged coma, local paresthesias, pneumonia, vocal cord paralysis, broken or fractured teeth, hepatitis and possible death.

4. I consent to the disposal by authorities of _____
_____ Hospital of any tissue or parts that
may be removed.

5. *I certify that I have read and understand* the foregoing and had the
contents of the foregoing explained to me and fully understand
the above consent for surgery; that I fully understand the procedure insofar as possible; and that the following points, among
others, have specifically been made clear to me regarding possible complications and unfavorable results:

   a. That the most common complications of abdominoplasty
   surgery are wound infection, dehiscence (to split open),
   hematoma, and necrosis (skin loss), and that these may occur.

   b. That deep leg phlebitis or pulmonary emboli may occur.

   c. That umbilical scar contracture may occur.

   d. That a scar revision may have to be performed on the incision
   line.

   e. I acknowledge that *no guarantee* or *assurance* has been made by
   the doctor above named to me with regard to the incision line
   result obtained and that readily visible scars after abdominoplasty are inevitable.

6. I further acknowledge that the usual risks and hazards of both
the surgical procedure and necessary anesthetic were made
known to me and that I accept full responsibility for these or any
other complication that may arise or result during the surgical
procedure(s), which is to be performed at my request according
to this consent and surgical permit for abdominoplasty. I further
acknowledge that all blanks or statements requiring insertion or
completion were filled in before I affixed my signature.

_____
(Signature of patient)

When patient is a minor or incompetent to
give consent:

_____
(Signature of person authorized to consent for patient)

_____
(Relationship to patient)

_____
(Witness)

_____
(Signature of patient's spouse)

Frederick M. Grazer, M.D.

Consent for Thighplasty

Patient _____ Age _____

A.M.

Date _____ Time P.M. _____ Place _____

1. I hereby authorize Dr. Frederick M. Grazer and whomever he may designate as his assistants to perform upon _____

   (State name of

   _____ the following operation(s):
   patient or "myself")

   and if any unforeseen condition arises in the course of this operation calling, in his judgment, for procedures in addition to or different from those contemplated, I further request and authorize him to do whatever he deems advisable and necessary in the circumstance.

2. I have been informed that the clinical outcome in my case does not only bear a relationship to the nature of the pathology (that is, the condition revealed, disclosed, or discovered by the procedure or procedures), but also bears a relationship to me insofar as there are individual variations of a physiological nature that influence recovery from the above described procedure(s) and that may or may not predispose to complications (see below). The nature, purpose, and risk of the operation and procedures and possible alternative methods of treatment and the possibility of complications have been explained fully to me. I acknowledge that no guarantee or assurance has been made as to the results that may be obtained.

3. I consent, authorize, and request the administration of such anesthetic or anesthetics as is deemed suitable by the physician-anesthetist who is an independent contractor and consultant. I fully understand that the physician-anesthetist will have full charge of the administration and maintenance of the general anesthetic and that this is an independent function from the operative procedure, and that Dr. Grazer has no responsibility for or direct control over the administration of the general anesthetic during the surgical procedure(s) and I have been fully informed of and understand that my exposure to anesthesia during the operation may result in adverse consequences, such as paralysis, coma or prolonged coma, local paresthesias, pneumo-

nia, vocal cord paralysis, broken or fractured teeth, hepatitis, and possible death.

4. I consent to the disposal by authorities of _____
_____Hospital of any tissue parts that may be removed.

5. *I certify that I have read and understand* the foregoing and had the contents of the foregoing explained to me and fully understand the above consent for surgery; that I fully understand the procedure insofar as possible, and that the following points, among others, have been specifically made clear to me regarding possible complications and unfavorable results:

   a. That the most common complications of thighplasty surgery are wound infection, hematoma, tissue loss, and fat necrosis (dissolution of fat).

   b. That there will be conspicuous scar deformity.

   c. I acknowledge that *no guarantee* or *assurance* has been made by the doctor to me with regard to the incision line results obtained and that readily visible scars after thighplasty are inevitable.

   d. That scar revisions may have to be performed on the incision lines.

6. I further acknowledge that the usual risks and hazards of both the surgical procedure(s) and necessary anesthetic were made known to me and that I accept full responsibility for these or any other complications that may arise or result during the surgical procedure(s), which is to be performed at my request according to this consent and surgical permit for thighplasty. I further acknowledge that all blanks or statements requiring insertion or completion were filled in before I affixed my signature.

_____
(Signature of patient)

When the patient is a minor or incompetent to give consent:

_____
(Signature of person authorized to consent for patient)

_____
(Relationship to patient)

_____
(Witness)

_____
(Signature of patient's spouse)

Index